T0146695

Secrets

of My

Vegan Kitchen

Secrets *of My* Vegan Kitchen

A Journey into Reversing My Diabetes without Medication

Nara Schuler

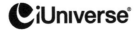

SECRETS OF MY VEGAN KITCHEN
A JOURNEY INTO REVERSING MY DIABETES WITHOUT MEDICATION

iUniverse books may be ordered through booksellers or by contacting:

iUniverse
1663 Liberty Drive
Bloomington, IN 47403
www.iuniverse.com
1-800-Authors (1-800-288-4677)

Because of the dynamic nature of the Internet, any web addresses or links contained in this book may have changed since publication and may no longer be valid. The views expressed in this work are solely those of the author and do not necessarily reflect the views of the publisher, and the publisher hereby disclaims any responsibility for them.

Any people depicted in stock imagery provided by Thinkstock are models, and such images are being used for illustrative purposes only. Certain stock imagery © Thinkstock.

ISBN: 978-1-5320-0179-6 (sc)
ISBN: 978-1-5320-0178-9 (e)

Library of Congress Control Number: 2016912676

Print information available on the last page.

iUniverse rev. date: 10/18/2016

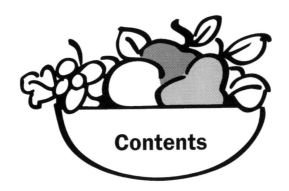

Contents

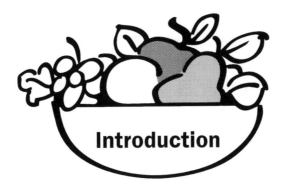

Introduction

Every time sitting at a dining table, we make a choice.
Please choose vegetarianism. Do it for the animals! Do it for
the environment and for the sake of your own health.
—Alec Baldwin

My journey on a plant-based diet started with my diagnosis of diabetes. I was so scared that I would be dependent on medications for the rest of my life that I had to find another way. Well, I found it. This book is about sharing my experience, and I hope to motivate many other people to take the same path and improve their health, if not completely reverse their diseases. Over the years, I have understood that to be healthy means not relying on taking any medications. Of course, you might have an occasional emergency situation where you need medication for one or two weeks, but taking it on a regular basis is just an excuse to eat and drink toxic foods. Some exceptions exist—I know—but if you are overweight, chances are you are not one of them.

I am not sure whether I will never have diabetes again in the future (maybe my genes are predisposed to it), but I am sure that I am taking the best possible care of my body. When my doctor offers me these fancy exams, such as a mammogram or colonoscopy, I wonder whether they will be able to prevent anything better than my good, whole foods, plant-based diet. I keep myself informed on the latest nutrition research, and I consistently read that the best way to prevent diseases is to eat an unprocessed diet with large amounts of vegetables, fruits, legumes, nuts, and seeds. While starting at an early age will give people a big advantage, it is never too late to start. Even people heavily dependent on medications will benefit from such changes, and they will feel reenergized and rejuvenated. Potentially, they will be able to reduce their medications and the accompanying side effects.

Our bodies are so incredibly resilient. Whenever we give them a chance, they flourish. There is no need for supplements, shakes, or any special formulas to achieve our most healthful state. There is no such thing as one super food; all vegetables, fruits, and grains are themselves super. Eating foods created by nature and prepared simply every day is all our bodies need.

The human body is very resourceful. It is like a complex machine that is capable of finding all it needs when fueled with the proper nutrition. Therefore, it is important to eliminate the foods that harm us, such as processed foods, which most often are from animal sources.

I hope to convince you to adopt this lifestyle change. I have added my daily recipes that are very simple and easy to prepare, to give you that push. Be kind to yourself, pay attention to what your body needs, and enjoy the journey.

Disclamer:

How Do We Decide What to Eat?

There are more than 70,000 edible plants on this planet
and some people choose to eat the flesh of animals.
—Pinterest.com

The real pleasure of eating can only be tasted, savored, or felt when we free our taste buds of toxic, addictive, caloricly empty foods. When we eat for addiction—which means we eat the same foods day after day at the first signal of hunger—we numb our palatal senses, and they become sensitive only to the foods we are used to eating. In order to free ourselves from this deficiency, we have to shift the way we eat. Only then are we free to make choices as to what we eat. The main reasons we choose particular foods are habit, convenience, societal (peer) pressure, and religion. Let's explore some of these factors.

Habit—Humans are creatures of habit; we feel comfortable when we do the same thing over and over again, day after day. This gives us a sense of comfort and power; the same happens with regard to our food. We tend to eat the same foods every day for breakfast, lunch, and dinner. Quite often, even when we go to different restaurants, we ask for the same dish. This is one of the reasons most restaurants tend to have quite similar options on their menus. Then there is that specialty option that is unique to a particular place, and when that is finally approved by the majority of consumers, it slowly becomes added to the menus of other establishments.

Convenience—We tend to eat what is easy and available. In today's society, it has become a trend to have instant meals, and because of a lack of time, we are often resigned to eating a bowl of cereal with milk for breakfast. Advertisements continuously make us believe that these foods are adequate for our nutritional needs. Fast-food restaurants filled with easy-to-make, cheap ingredients have also become very convenient, with an emphasis on taste rather than nutrition. It became easy for us to adopt this way of eating. On top of that, big companies consistently advertise the benefits of eating their food and the convenience of not having to prepare it.

Societal Pressure—It is very interesting to observe that people will make a big effort to fit into a group. We have the need to be approved of by the people around us, and choosing to eat and drink the same things creates a bond among people. How many times do you feel you just can't drink another cup of coffee but your friend wants to have one and invites you? You drink it just to visit with your friend. Or how many times do you accept that extra chocolate bar knowing that it will ruin your diet but your coworker offers you one and you can't resist? Or when you are paying your bill at a restaurant and they give you candies and you eat them because that is the "right" thing to do? Start standing up for your health, and you will feel how much pressure there is to eat the standard junk diet.

Religion—This is a reason that is ingrained in many people, and they either will or will not eat certain foods because they believe it will impact their spirituality.

We are living in a society where a large number of us act in an automated way. People seem to be hypnotized to behave in a certain manner. Not many of us stop to think about what is best for ourselves. People do what others do just to be one of the group.

Let's start looking at food. Why do people eat? One would say because they are hungry, but I would say that they are far from hungry. I would even venture to say that, in our society, most people don't even feel hungry sometimes, yet they eat anyway. The society where I am living right now in North America is the most overfed society in the world, yet many of us are undernourished and possibly overweight (J. Fuhrman 2011).

So the first concept here is that overeating has nothing to do with being well nourished. I was a culprit of following a standard Western diet for more than forty years, but when I was told by my doctor that I would need to take medication for the rest of my life, I decided to take another look at what I was eating. This situation has made an enormous impact in my life. It was hard at the beginning, but the results came so fast and so consistently that it seems impossible for me now not to share this experience with others.

We need to eat nutritious foods that will guarantee us a good state of health and allow us to remain healthy as we age. However, most of us have been convinced that nutritious foods are not tasty, which is far from the truth.

Whenever I talk with people about this subject, I have the impression that everyone is aware of the differences between eating for health and eating junk. So why is it so hard to change from a junky diet to a healthy one? If people consciously know these differences, why do they continue to overeat food that is lacking in nutrition?

The answer to that question lies partially in TV commercials, in restaurant preparations, in the industrialization of cheap food, and in an illusion of pleasure that is overpromoted. Very few of us are strong enough to admit that such pleasure is often transient and lacking in satisfaction. However, when I look around and observe what people are eating and how they eat it, I am surprised at how sturdy the human body is. Considering the amount of junk people ingest on a regular basis day after day, year after year, it seems obvious that we should be a very, very sick society. That is what we are becoming more and more.

One of the first things that amazes me is seeing the number of people who cannot eat a meal without animal products. They truly believe they will be lacking in protein and nutrition. There is a deep-rooted belief that people need to ingest enormous portions of fat and protein and huge quantities of highly processed grains in the form of breads or cereal in many of their meals, with the addition of sugar or salt, to make the flavor stronger. To make things even worse, food portions nowadays are larger than ever before, and we all order them in combos to save a few dollars. It should come as no surprise that a lower quality of life is ahead. In a desperate attempt at healthful eating, some people top up the meal with one slice of tomato or a lettuce leaf. As if this addition would make a difference in the nutrition content of the meal! To compliment their meals, most people also drink large amounts of soda pop or sweetened juices.

This is insane!

Chapter 2

My Family's Eating Habits

Nothing will benefit human health and increase chances for survival
of life on Earth as much as the evolution to a vegetarian diet.
—Albert Einstein

I was born into a family where my parents had completely different
views of dietary needs. My father was always looking into healthy
ways of eating, and starting in his thirties, he adopted a raw fruit diet
for a week each year. When I was a child, my father was already inclined
to avoid animal products, but this was an extreme idea for those days; and
my mother, for years, would add a leg of chicken when cooking his beans
and remove it just before he could discover what she had done.

My mother used to believe my father would not have enough energy if
that chicken leg was not in his food. He did not eat completely healthfully
because he didn't like vegetables very much, which, from my point of view
and that of much of the current research (T. C. Campbell 2004), are the
main pillars of a healthy diet. However, the way my father ate at least
prevented him from eating damaging food throughout his life. He usually
ate whole seasonal food comprised mostly of legumes, nuts, and fruits.
He passed at eighty-eight. Although his brain was very alert, he had some
motor difficulties at the end, which caused depression; that caused him
to give up on life. My mother, on the other hand, was able to eat as much

as she wanted and anything available. The good news for her was that she loved beans, fruits, and vegetables as well.

During my teenage years, my mother opened a bakery and a fast-food restaurant. I think that it was from that moment on that I became addicted to junk food. Until then, I was quite removed from harmful foods because we were fortunate not to have access to soda pop; canned, processed food; and other junk. Most of what we ate was real, healthy, organically grown food. I believe that this start helped me to create a foundation of healthy cells and strength in my body.

In the late '70s, one of my older sisters became a vegetarian, and she was quite strict for some years. I used to like to go to her house to eat. It was different from what I had at home, but it was very tasty: lots of vegetables, lightly cooked, and absolutely no processed foods. She did not overcook her greens, and I think that was her biggest cooking secret. She allowed them to reach their peak flavor and then served them immediately. At that time, I was young and healthy, and I didn't think I needed to change my diet. From my point of view, the diet I was eating was serving me well. I put on about twenty pounds during my twenties and thirties, but so did everyone else, and I just enjoyed eating whatever I wanted: lots of meat, bread, pop (mostly diet), ice cream, a little bit of salad—just because, like everyone else in the world, I thought that one lettuce leaf, one slice of tomato, and one broccoli stem would make me healthy.

In my forties, I started to have some health problems here and there, but so did everyone else. Who out there does not take a pain pill or two each day? Who does not get a sore throat and a cold once or twice a year? I believed it was just the way we all aged. My weight continued to increase. In my late forties, I remember expressing my concerns about my increasing weight to my family doctor. He told me that I was not obese, I was just a little overweight and there was nothing to worry about because I was quite healthy compared to everyone else. So I continued to eat as I pleased, whatever everyone else ate, and the weight and pounds continued piling up year after year.

It was in my early fifties when the weight started to bother me. I weighed 249 pounds while my ideal weight was 145. You can figure out that there were almost two of me in one body. On top of having so much more fat in my body than I needed, I started having many medical problems.

Chapter 3

Social Influences on My Food Choices

When diet is wrong, medicine is of no use. When
diet is correct, medicine is of no need.
—Ayurvedic proverb

This book is not a medical prescription and does not replace any medical advice. If you have health issues, you should consult your physician and discuss your best alternative with him/her. However, I hope the story in this book will make each of you stop and think about your own health issues and research alternatives, all the while discussing your condition with your health-care professional. Do not go blindly to an appointment with a health practitioner and let another person make such important decisions for you.

Often in our society, we are politely bullied into doing what a health-care professional suggests. When we go to a medical appointment, we are normally fragile and anxious to talk about how we feel. Health-care professionals are trained to treat symptoms, and most of the time, this is not a cure, even though we are led to think it is. While there are cures out there for many health problems, they may not be magic wands. Quite often a real cure requires a lot of lifestyle changes. Unfortunatly the importance of these lifestyle changes are not necessarily recommended or explained by most physicians.

Therefore, if you have a diagnosis, take a few days to research your illness. What causes it? How do other people deal with it? Find out how many patients your doctor has treated and what happened to them after a year of treatment and longer. Ask questions. Today it is so easy to go on the Internet and find thousands of people with the same diagnosis. Learn how they are doing and, most important, find out the ones whose symptoms have disappeared and how they have addressed it.

This was my approach, and I could not be happier with my decision. I may or may not have cured my type 2 diabetes, but I can guarantee you that five years after being diagnosed, I am considered by any medical test to be nondiabetic. I have not taken any medication during these five years. If, on the other hand, I had allowed my doctor to give me the traditional treatment for type 2 diabetes, I doubt I would be in such good health at this moment. I would probably be increasing the amount of pharmaceutical drugs and may be even starting insulin injections like so many others do.

Whether or not you are a professional health practitioner, you know yourself and your own body better than anyone else, and you have an obligation to look out for what is best for you.

My experience has proven to me that there is nothing more important than eating a healthy diet. When one wants to restore health, it is imperative to get rid of all junk food. That is the purpose of this book: to let you know that a person of fifty-one years of age, very addicted to all sorts of unhealthy food, obese, and diagnosed with type 2 diabetes, can be transformed into a healthy fifty-two-year-old with many more years to come without any medication. I am at close to my ideal body weight without even trying and, by all accounts, I look ten years younger. Eating a highly nutritious diet composed of whole, plant-based foods and eliminating all highly processed food was, for me, the real source of youth.

Chapter 4

I Recognized I Was Sick

Collectively the media; the meat, oil, and dairy industries; most
prominent chefs and cookbook authors; and our own government
are not presenting accurate advice about the healthiest way to eat.
—Caldwell Esselstyn Jr.

In February 2009, I started to notice that my vision was sometimes
becoming blurry. One day I was driving at dusk, and I noticed I could
not read the street signs just a few feet away. I started worrying about
my vision. My blood pressure was around 160/120, but I cannot say I felt
the effects of it, at least not at a conscious level. I went to see an eye doctor.
After he tested my eyesight, he prescribed glasses and told me to talk to
my family doctor. I remember that while I was looking for a pair of glasses
at the store, I happened to notice my image in the mirror and thought
that I was looking at my grandma's face. I was appalled. My grandmother
was seventy-two when I was born, so guess how old she was when I had
memories of her; and I had just turned fifty-one. I became worried, but
not enough to take any action yet. I bought the eyeglasses but did not book
an appointment with a physician. I continued with my life eating a pretty
standard Western diet, which included meat, burgers, bread, cheese, milk,
potatoes, cookies, coffee, diet sodas, and so on. I ate a few vegetables—just
enough to tell everyone that I ate them.

A few months after I acquired my eyeglasses in the winter of 2009, I started having urinary infections. Since I am more prone to taking natural medications, I started drinking lots of cranberry juice. The infections receded for a while but returned a couple of months later, around spring of 2010. Finally, in September of that year, I concluded I needed help from my physician to get rid of such recurring infections, and I booked an appointment to see him. I took a urine sample with me because I thought they would need to examine it. To my surprise, he told me I was diabetic. My blood sugar was 14.4 mmoL/L, and I was fasting at that moment. They made such a strong point of me being diabetic that my doctor wanted me to start taking medication immediately.

Unfortunately, *getting older* is a synonym for getting sicker. It is sad to think that our society only values new things. Older people have made mistakes and, as a result, have become sick, but younger ones will make those same mistakes. Let's just give them time!

One of the biggest mistakes we make is to believe that our health is in someone else's hands and that a container of pills holds the cure. Another one is believing that we are immune to diseases because our bodies were functioning well when we were young. I have held both of those beliefs for years, as have many other people. To some extent, I feel that I was fortunate to have had two medical experiences that awakened me from the belief that the only way to find a cure is through pharmaceutical drugs. While the amazing advances in medicine are important, and there is a place for them in acute and emergency situations, chronic conditions should first be addressed by exploring nutritional interventions. Our first option for chronic disease should always be to give our bodies the opportunity to heal themselves by removing all toxic foods, such as highly processed foods and foods from animal sources, while at the same time replenishing our bodies with large quantities of a variety of whole plants, such as vegetables, legumes, whole grains, and fruits, which are high in nutrients.

When my father died, I became deeply depressed for about a year. I was so devastated that my doctor suggested that I should start on antidepression medication. I was a little reluctant at first because I was afraid of becoming addicted to it. However, my doctor convinced me to take it with the following words: "Let's think of it as a nondefined period of time." So I agreed and started taking the drug. I thought at the time that those words meant that I would be taking the medication for a short period of time, while I was very depressed. I believed that I would eventually come out of it because I would feel better and be cured. Over the years, I realized that such an assumption was completely incorrect.

At the beginning, the medication did wonders for me. I became happy within a few weeks. I felt no side effects, and life was great. It was only after a year or two that I started feeling that the medication was not treating my depressive state anymore, and I went back to my doctor for a change in my prescription. Does this sound familiar? Time continued to pass, and I kept on going to my doctor's office every three months to get a refill for my pills. Five years passed, and I was asked to go for a cardiogram. The cardiologist told me that my heart was doing fine, but I was possibly having side effects from my depression medication. This cardiologist advised me to talk to my family doctor and ask him to reduce the dosage of my depression med. I followed this recommendation, but my family doctor told me I needed to continue to take an antidepressant or I would be in danger of having serious consequences. I trusted him and accepted his recommendation and continued taking the prescription.

I believe that my family doctor has always acted in my best interests; however, I think that the way the medical system is structured makes it very difficult for physicians to understand that the help of medications should be only temporary. Doctors should lead patients to a cure, not just alleviate symptoms, which intensifies the risk of other diseases through increased dosages of medication. Pharmaceuticals should be used in emergencies or in acute crises and should not be regarded as a continuous treatment to suppress symptoms. A cure is possible when the true cause is faced and only when the patient is completely involved in addressing it. Doctors have an obligation to use their knowledge to educate their patients in what they need to do to accomplish a cure.

Another huge problem is that our society believes that cures come from outside the body rather than from within. There is an acceptance that magic pills will bring back health, and this continues to be conveniently advertised by big pharma. To some extent, the relief of a symptom feels like a cure because the discomfort is relieved and we all enjoy that extended period of time that lasts between four and twelve hours. I understand ... we become addicted to feeling good.

The amazing truth is that such relief can be permanent for many patients if they become seriously involved in making their cure happen. Difficult changes need to be made, but they are worth it. I used to think that I should believe in my doctor because he had a medical degree. I realized later that even though doctors have a more comprehensive understanding of disease and they can explain the seriousness of some illnesses, only we can really appreciate the nature of our symptoms and take real steps back to good health. We know more about ourselves than anyone else. There are many conditions where a knowledgeable doctor will guide patients in finding the proper way to address their health problem, without the need to force medications down their throats. Our physicians should encourage us to find a diet that will lead to a cure or at least minimize our dependence on medications.

As time passed, I started having more side effects from my antidepressants, like bloating, for which my doctor prescribed a mild medication. This increased not only my already high blood pressure but also my obesity. I did not want to keep increasing the number of medications, and, for this reason, I decided to experiment with cutting out all my medications cold turkey. I know this is a dangerous thing to do, and I am not recommending anyone do this without first consulting a health care professional. I am simply telling you what I did. It might not have been the smartest thing to do, but I did it anyway. I did this before I changed my diet, because I was already scared of never getting off my meds.

There are medical professionals out there who are capable of caring for their patients without resorting to medications, and this is the type of advice we all should be getting. Since I did not get that advice, I made my own decision and stuck to it. It was a very crazy time. I felt as though I was walking on clouds for a week or two. I heard metallic sounds inside my brain bouncing from one side to the other. In the first two days, the sounds were stronger and more frequent, but, as the days went by, the sounds became weaker until I could not hear them anymore. I overcame my withdrawal symptoms, and I do not regret making this decision and assuming the risk. I would say that either I am very strong or my depression wasn't as damaging as the pharmaceutical companies made me believe. Again, please do not attempt to do this without help from a medical doctor.

During this time, I was already obese and completely addicted to junk food and sweet drinks and, most important, I could not see the danger of this addiction. Of course my doctor gave me some advice that I should eat better, as all health practitioners always do, but he failed to emphasize the importance of such nutritional change. At that time, I could not understand the future consequences of my eating habits. But time went on, and fat continued to store up in my body. I started to have some weird feelings. My distance vision seemed to go black from time to time, my blood pressure was as high as 160/120, and I felt very tired climbing stairs. I developed sleep apnea, urinary infections, and body inflamation. It took me a couple of months of such miserable sensations before I decided to go see my doctor, at which time I was diagnosed with type 2 diabetes.

I did not like that diagnosis, mainly because my doctor told me I had to start taking pills for an undetermined time. It was his expression, "undetermined time," that made something inside me change. Hearing those words reminded me of my previous experience with the antidepressants and triggered an image of myself going from one medication to a stronger one, adding more and more medications and having increased side effects that would lead to more medications. I thought to myself, *There has to be a better way to treat diabetes.* I declined my doctors offer on the spot.

When I returned home, I immediately started researching diabetes. After reading several articles, I found one that seemed to bring hope of a cure. This is what I want to share with you: a way we can actively participate in reversing or curing many of our health problems with food and happiness.

I absolutely hate the idea of becoming dependent on anything or anyone. I thought of this at that moment when my doctor told me that my genes had caused my diabetes and that I would have to take drugs forever. In my mind, I could see myself taking several other drugs, as many people do in our society. At that moment, I said to myself, *No! I do not want this!* I thought, *There has to be a way that I can continue to be free from the pharmaceutical companies.*

That day changed my life. I reflected upon everything my father used to say about food. I reflected on what my sisters had told me about food, their experiences and the effects on their health. I made a vow to take care of myself. I decided that I am the one who knows my body better than anyone else. I decided that I should take responsibility for what was going on with me and my body, instead of giving control to someone who is very nice to me when I show up at his office once or twice a year for thirty minutes.

At that moment, I started my research for a cure, first from the diabetes and, later, for my addiction to food. Yes, an addiction to food that I am still battling even though I suspect that I eat healthier than 90 percent of people. I still eat too much food as I have not yet reached my ideal weight. I want to tell you this now because I want you all to know that those two things are different. I was able to cure my diabetes and many other health issues in spite of still being addicted to food. I continue to work on this problem, and I am sure, eventually, I will be free of this addiction too.

In the days after this diabetes verdict, I read as much as I could about diabetes, and I came across Dr. Joel Fuhrman's book *Eat to Live*. At that moment, what I read made sense, and I decided to give it a try. I gave myself a three-month window of opportunity to try his diet and check with my doctor to see if anything had changed in my body. I told myself that if no improvement happened in that period, I would be resigned to my doctor's advice and surrender myself to the medical and pharmaceutical industries.

In the first few days, I got rid of all foods that I had at home or in my diet that Dr. Fuhrman classified as unhealthy. That meant no more sugar or sweeteners, alcohol, highly processed flours, meat, milk, or dairy. I also discarded less damaging ones, such as starchy roots and flours, and any animal products. I confess I felt sorry for myself because I had to give up so many of my favorite foods. But I looked at Dr. Fuhrman's food pyramid and made a decision that whatever I was going to eat would have to belong on one of the three lowest rows. I could make any combination of foods from those categories, but I was limited to those three rows (vegetables, fruits, legumes, seeds, and nuts). Once I planted this idea in my mind, I started to explore a huge range of options. To my surprise, I was able to create tasty food. I started giving myself credit for finding out about this. Within a couple of days, I started to feel fortunate that there were so many food options available to me. I confess also that, at the beginning, I did not really like the taste of these new foods, but I felt comfort in knowing that at least this was an option to becoming less dependent on doctors and pharmacies. This was really important to me.

Little by little, I started to like my new diet, but more important than liking the taste of it, I was noticing changes in the way I felt. My diet consisted of a vegetable smoothie in the morning, a bowl of beans with steamed vegetables for lunch, and a soup made from the leftovers for dinner. I also included a cup of freshly made vegetable juices every night as a treat. I started making my food in a way that looked appealing to my eyes. I made a point of placing the food in nice dishes, decorating the table with a beautiful table cloth, and serving the juices in clear crystal glasses so I could appreciate the tonality of the colors. That step made me look forward to what I would create next and what would be attractive to others when they looked at my food. Every day, someone from my family wanted to try my food and, even though they were still eating their regular standard Western diet, they began to try what I was eating. And they liked it too. This was an important step in changing my diet.

I used to take over-the-counter painkillers for frequent pain in my body—sometimes headaches, other times pain in my hips, legs, stomach, and so on. As I became more regular with the new diet, my need for painkillers decreased accordingly. In the first week after I changed my diet, I had night sweats. I remember once I woke up in the middle of the night and

I felt a sort of an explosion in my liver area. It was as though a match had lighted a propane tank in there, and a second later, my body was completely wet from head to toe. I had to wake up my husband and completely change our bedsheets and clothes. I was very afraid that night, but I felt some relief in my body, and I got back into a deep sleep.

During the first three or four weeks of this new diet, I felt night sweats often. The strongest one was the first, but I had many other episodes, and I confess, I did feel scared. Part of me wanted to book an appointment with my doctor and ask him if this was normal, but deep inside, I knew that he would know less than I did about it since he did not show any interest in my dietary changes. I decided to trust my instincts and stay on the plan for the three-month tryout while giving my body the opportunity to heal itself. As the weeks went by, I needed fewer painkillers. My eyesight improved, and I shed pound after pound. I was feeling better and better. I used to have pain in my hips during the night while sleeping, which used to wake me up from time to time. Within a couple of weeks, that pain became scarcer and scarer. It was a weird feeling. I knew the pain would not come back.

When I went back to my doctor's office after the three-month trial period of my new dietary regimen, we redid my blood test. He was surprised to see that all my blood functions were back to normal ranges, including my blood sugar levels.

He considered me free from type 2 diabetes at that time, and it has stayed that way since. Obviously, if I ever go back to eating the way I did before, the problem will recur. Therefore, this dietary change is really a life change and has to be faced accordingly.

Getting Information on Food Choices and Health

Do the best you can until you know better. Then
when you know better, do better.
—Maya Angelou

I started reading other authors on the subject of healthy eating, and I became convinced that our society is totally wrong and brainwashed in regard to what is accepted as healthy. People overeat constantly and, as if this is not enough, people overeat bad quality food. No wonder the world is now facing a crisis of obesity and chronic diseases.

I know there is a huge volume of literature by well-qualified doctors and researchers explaining the need for diet changes. I am neither a doctor nor a researcher; however, I have had the sense to stop the insanity I was living and start paying attention to my own needs. I was able to implement what was best for me.

While writing these pages, it is my intention to explain simple and inexpensive changes we can make on a daily basis to protect ourselves from illness and painful suffering. Unfortunately, many people in our society have already accepted that, after fifty years of age, everyone will need to take a wide variety of medications every day. We see this in movies, we hear this from our doctors, we help our family members take pills, and we continuously see this in TV commercials. It is scary that drug commercials list several dangerous side effects from medications and yet people still believe it is better to take them instead of adopting simple changes to their diets.

Based on my personal experience, I can guarantee you that once you experiment and feel the pleasures of your body healing and rejuvenating, you will not want to go back to eating an unhealthy diet and camouflaging your symptoms with drugs.

I am advocating for a healthier lifestyle, not a new diet.

Studies show a huge growth in the number of sick people, the vast majority of whom suffer from chronic diseases that afflict all groups (D. Fuhrman 2005). Today, these diseases include heart disease, type 2 diabetes, obesity, osteoporosis, and breast, colon, and prostate cancer. Many of these conditions can be prevented by eating the right foods and avoiding the toxic ones. Some of them can even be reversed, as has been proved by many physicians (T. C. Campbell 2004). Why do people continue to promote eating a standard American diet? Why do people choose to undergo life-threatening surgeries instead of making simple dietary changes?

We need to make use of the extensive information gleaned from research and come to our own conclusions. It is important to make a judgment on how we want to be living ten, twenty, thirty years from now. What we ingest today will either enhance or restrict our capabilities in the future.

When we hear the saying "We are what we eat," we expect results to show the very next day. In reality, the accumulation of toxins from a standard American diet will only surface within a couple of years because of the resilience of our bodies. That could be one of the reasons we disregard the signs of disease. We do not believe it will happen to us. Remarkably, however, when we change our diet to a whole foods, plant-based one, our bodies start to show a difference within a couple of weeks. This has been experienced by the testimonials of thousands of patients from Dr. Fuhrman (Success Stories n.d.), and other physicians, including me.

Vitamins, minerals, macro and micronutrients, proteins, fats, and also toxins accumulate in our bodies over time. What we choose to provide our cells with will be retained and will define how our bodies function.

If you eat a standard American diet, you should reflect on how many contaminants your body ingests day after day. While our bodies are able to eliminate some of these toxins, others will be accumulated continuously. Years and years of daily toxin accumulation will turn into disease. "What diseases?" one would ask. That will depend on our genes. Here, genes can define variances in our health. Our genetics will define the triggers to different illnesses after a significant amount of saturation in our bodies (Peto 1981). However, maintaining a healthy, nutrition-filled diet will tend to keep genetic triggers dormant (T. C. Campbell 2004). It is quite hard for some of us to accept this concept as nutrition is still a new science.

As I have mentioned before, I believe you are the only person who can decide how you want to live as you age. There is a popular belief that being old and being sick are synonymous this is not necessarily the case. One can age and still be healthy and have a very rewarding and pleasant life. The crazy tyranny of the popular diet is starting to be reflected in younger and younger people as they bear the brunt of diet-related diseases. Disease is not a result of growing older but a syndrome of bad food choices.

The following paragraphs are an excerpt from Fuhrman's *Eat to Live,* and they summarize what I have experienced since I changed my diet:

> For most people, illness means putting their fate in the hands of doctors and complying with their recommendations— recommendations that typically involve taking drugs for the rest of their lives while they watch their health gradually deteriorate. People are completely unaware that most illnesses are self-induced and can be reversed with aggressive nutritional methods.

Both patients and physicians act as though everyone's medical problems are genetic or assumed to be the normal consequence of aging. They believe that chronic illness is just what we all must expect. Unfortunately, the medical-pharmaceutical business has encouraged people to believe that health problems are hereditary and that we need to swallow poisons to defeat our genes. This is almost always untrue. We all have genetic weaknesses, but those weaknesses never get a chance to express themselves until we abuse our body with many, many years of mistreatment. Never forget, 99 percent of your genes are programmed to keep you healthy. The problem is that we never let them do their job. (J. Fuhrman 2011)

In the body of literature available on this subject, several authors and experts differ a little here and there; however they all promote and agree that a minimally processed, plant-based diet with the infrequent inclusion of an animal product is the most healthful to us humans.

Most doctors agree that highly processed grains, sugar, and animal products create and promote the growth of diseases, the same ones that are becoming epidemic in the United States, Canada, Europe, and so many countries around the world.

Disease is created by the lack of good nutrition. Fascinatingly, it is never too late to start eating more healthfully. Start today! Eliminate all junk food. Eliminate empty calorie foods from your diet. Eat large amounts of vegetables, fruits, and legumes. You will feel the difference in your own body within a couple of weeks. If you fall off the wagon, do not worry; get back on track at the next meal.

It feels amazing not to have that hip pain. It feels amazing to be able to get up from a chair and not hear and feel a cracking sound in the knee, to be able to read a street sign from a distance without the need of glasses, to have a desire to go for a walk, to exercise and live life again. We forget about these simple pleasures once we get addicted to food pleasures. We grow accustomed to living with the odd ache or pain that quietly grows worse. But as soon as we regain these freedoms, we will not want to exchange them for any pleasure coming from unhealthy foods. There is no cake that can compete with a pain-free hip; there is no barbecue pleasure that can replace the relief of a healthy bowel movement; there is no milk chocolate that can replace the relief of breathing an unobstructed breath of air.

When I talk to people about these feelings, it always surprises me to hear that people think they cannot implement such changes in their diet. I always wonder why. Does a piece of cake mean more to this person than their health? What is in a slice of bread that makes it more important than a pain-free belly? What is it in a plate of ribs, a hamburger, a portion of french fries? It has to do with taste, but also with emotional attachments, nostalgia, and social pressure.

Chapter 6

Making Choices

People may hate you for being different and not
living by society's standards but deep down, they
wish they had the courage to do the same.
—anonymous

A huge problem with addressing changing eating habits is that there is so much confusing information about food that sometimes it becomes difficult to find credible sources. Many medical or other health institutions are still attached to previously formed ideas that were rooted in the financial investment of industries that profess to have people's best interests at heart but really don't.

A typical example is the popular notion that we quench thirst with a can of pop instead of a pure, simple glass of water. When I was a child, we used to have water available at every meal, and we would just grab a cup of tap water when thirsty. How many of us still do this? As I was growing up, it became a status symbol to have pop when people would come for a visit. Then it was in fashion to have pop for children on their birthdays. (What better way to get people addicted to something than to entice them at their most nostalgic, childhood moments!) Today, people automatically reach for a pop when they're thirsty. While watching movies and commercials, in which actors grab a can from a pop machine to quench their thirst, we have become used to the idea that this is the right way to satiate thirst. We do not realize that every time we open a pop and drink that liquid, our bodies become more acidic. It happens little by little over the years. Most of us don't know that a can of pop has a pH level of 2.5 (which is highly acidic), and some of us who do know don't care because we are somehow convinced that this is acceptable.

Few of us will worry that our bodies continually strive to maintain a normal pH balance between 7.3 and 7.45. This pH level is important because when we are slightly alkaline, our body's metabolic, enzymatic, immunologic, and repair mechanisms are able to perform at their best. PH levels are measured on a logarithmic scale. It means, in simple words, that to move from a level of 2.5 to 3.5, the body needs increase alkalization 10 times—from 3.5 to 4.5 another 10 times. You can see how this is going to end to reach a level of 7.5, right? 10 by 10 by 10 by 10 by 10, which means 100,000 times alkalization improvement. This implies that to neutralize the effects of consuming one can of pop, we would need to drink the equivalent of thirty-two cans of good-quality water to return our body pH to an acceptable level (between 7.3 and 7.45) (Ribeiro 2013).

Think for a second: How many cans of pop do you drink every day? This simple exercise easily illustrates just how strong our bodies are and how much toxic abuse we can be exposed to before our health starts to irreversibly deteriorate. It is amazing that we can still function perfectly for some years before we start to feel the effects of the toxic waste we have allowed to enter our bodies. However, if you are interested in preparing for a bright future in which your body will perform optimally later in your life, you will have to address your diet and lifestyle choices now. An acidic body impacts our overall health. It creates the perfect condition for inflammation and hormonal imbalances, and it is the backdrop for uric acid accumulation and retention of toxic minerals, all the while inhibiting our abilities to absorb and retain vitamins and minerals. There is a lot of literature available on this subject if you want to explore more.

Unfortunately, the routine consumption of large amounts of pop is only one of our society's bad habits. Our problems do not end there. For instance, we also have the habit of eating the same foods every day, cooked and seasoned the same way. Even when eating a nutritious diet, this kind of regularity might lead to lack of nutrients over time. Now, imagine if the ingredients in your food are already acidic and bad for you. While eating the same foods every day might be easier for some people, it may not serve our best nutritional interests. Preparing and serving the same foods every day is certainly easier and more economical for commercial establishments. It is simpler for stores and restaurants to prepare and plan their sales, to track their stock, and to keep costs and staff education to a minimum. This might be our reward for preparing the very same recipe from one meal to the next every single day of our lives.

Having an assortment of food ingredients cooked in a variety of ways is always better. Healthy eating demands a multiplicity of foods, colors, flavors, and texture. We are so lucky! Never in human history has humankind had such an assortment of foods available at the corner store. In our supermarkets, most of us enjoy a huge selection of fruits and vegetables that come from several parts of the world. These imports can be used in many different ways to embrace dishes that would please the most sophisticated culinary palate, day after day, without repeating a recipe for a long period of time. Eating this way would uncover the potential for keeping us healthy, without the need for medicinal supplements.

The most common objection I hear about improving one's diet is that it takes more time to cook this way. Nonsense! A great dish can be as complicated or as simple as one wishes. Some days I spend less than fifteen minutes preparing our food; other days I spend hours. It all depends on how sophisticated I want my meals to be. I would dare to state that the simpler the preparation of these natural ingredients, the better it is for our health.

Most days I cook my beans from scratch. I simmer them for two to three hours on low heat. However, when I do not have time, I open a can of beans, steam a bunch of precut frozen vegetables, and make a simple salad with lettuce, tomato, onions, a handful of almonds, and sunflower seeds. When I want to impress a friend, I might make a vegetable lasagna, a meatless "meat" pie, a stuffed pumpkin, or another savory dish, the recipe for which can be easily found on the Internet or in vegetarian cookbooks.

In terms of cost, there is also a huge difference in eating a healthy diet. It is cheaper, believe it or not. Processed food can be quite expensive, and nature-made food is still quite accessible. When you switch to natural, whole, plant-based food, you will be surprised at the savings in your grocery bill, even if you decide to buy organic.

However, the real benefit is that you become healthier. This is where the huge savings are, but we are not used to including these costs when planning our weekly budget. We have a tendency to believe that we will never need medications, treatments, medical equipment, insurance, and so forth. In reducing disease and pain, we are also eliminating the need for medical and pharmaceutical interventions and their overheads. It makes sense to look into all aspects of dietary changes: economic, ecological, psychological, and the like. While feeling better is the main goal, saving money is a welcome side effect.

Unfortunately for many of us, this revelation comes only after we are faced with the reality of lack of mobility, constant pain, or other medical threats. Even more unfortunate is that some people will never agree to change their diet and will resign themselves to a miserable, painful life and continue suffering just for the pleasure of eating familiar foods. Their sense of food nostalgia and familiarity is strong enough to fight diet change or food experimentation, simple measures that could bring so much benefit.

By now, you already know that I truly believe that eating a diet composed of whole, plant-based foods can completely eradicate or reverse many diseases, and that part of the problem in implementing this practice is that only a few members of the medical community believe in it.

When I had a diagnosis of type 2 diabetes, my doctor offered me the standard solution: indefinite use of blood-sugar-lowering pills, starting immediately, with a moderate change in my diet. I was furious. He said that diabetes was in my genes. I said, "No way! I do not want to be sick! I will not be sick!" After arguing with my doctor about my treatment, I bargained with him to give me three months to make my transformation. I decided to look into an alternative approach and, if I didn't find it, I would comply with what he was suggesting.

That is when my quest for good health began. I frantically went onto the Internet and looked for a medical approach to reverse my diagnosis … and I found it. I read all I could about diabetes and radically modified my diet. Imagine my doctor's surprise when he saw my blood test results after three months! I had reversed the condition that he had diagnosed, and since then, I have not needed to take a single medication. If you think I am the only one, I suggest you look at several websites and read the testimonials of many patients who have had the same results; I recommend that you start with Dr. Fuhrman's website. I am not being paid—nor have I been asked to promote his site here; I am only telling you the truth of what has happened to me.

Chapter 7

Science, Myths, and Food

If you do not have time to take care of your health now, you will have to find time to take care of your disease in the future.
—Dr. Joel Fuhrman

I cannot tell you what to eat or what diet is going to be the best for you. That is a personal decision. I can only tell you that if you decide to give your body a chance, choose to eat a diet high in nutrients, and eliminate all junk and foods with empty calories, your body will respond and reverse most of the diseases it has been accumulating over the years. Some of you will need the help of your physicians because it becomes a little trickier if you are already being medicated, but it can still be done. It is simple: dramatically increase the amount of vegetables, fruits, and legumes in your diet on a daily basis, and eliminate all processed food and drinks. There is no need for magic potions or super foods.

Often when I say this to people, they think they just need to add vegetables and fruits or salads to their meals; however, only adding whole and plant-based foods to your diet is not enough. It is the replacement of processed foods with vegetables, fruits, and legumes that will make the difference. I now eat about one pound of raw vegetables and one pound of cooked vegetables every day. I complement my diet with fresh fruit, beans, and seeds or nuts. I season my food with natural lime or lemon juice, pineapple, herbs, or dry peppers. I do not use salt or oil when preparing my meals. Having plant-based ingredients in all my dishes is enough to make me feel satisfied, and it tastes delicious. Plus, I am healthier today than I was ten years ago.

If your physician tells you that it is not possible to change your diet so radically, it might be better to look for another physician who is more informed and aware of the influence nutrition has on our health. Fortunately, nowadays there is an increasing number of doctors out there who have a nutritional background and favor diet improvement over medication. They choose the best option for their patients so they can achieve a quality lifestyle in later years.

Dr. Fuhrman says, "A cure for cancer has already been found: eat more vegetables!" Sadly, very few of us are willing to accept this truth. A large number of people don't want to change their poor eating habits. They don't want to let go of highly processed food, sugars, and animal products. They think their meals will lose taste and flavor. My experience has been exactly the opposite. The more I explore vegetables and fruits, the more amazing are the tastes and flavors in my life.

In the paragraph that follows, I will describe a little bit of the work of pioneering medical professionals in the field of nutrition. If you are interested in reading more about their work, I made a list below of the physicians and authors who have inspired me on this journey:

- Joel Fuhrman, MD
- Caldwell Esselstyn Jr., MD
- John A. McDougall, MD
- Neal Barnard, MD
- Thomas Campbell MD
- Michael Klaper, MD
- T. Colin Campbell
- Michael Greger, MD

Dr. Joel Fuhrman, in his books *Eat to Live*, *Super Immunity*, *The End of Diabetes*, and so on, recommends eating one pound of raw vegetables and one pound of cooked vegetables, plus fruits, beans, and healthy fats (such as avocado, nuts, and seeds) every day. This should account for at least 90 percent of your daily food intake. Such a recommendation, when followed over a short period of time—for example, just three weeks—is enough to supply most of the nutrients our bodies need and will help stop cravings for junk food. The remaining 10 percent of our daily meals could consist of grains, fish, eggs, and so forth, but preferably whole foods that are plant based.

Plant-based whole foods are attractive and have an amazing taste. Try to be unbiased and open to new experiences. Just because you have tried broccoli before and didn't like it doesn't mean all broccoli out there will taste the same.

Our perception of taste is very interesting because once we cleanse our taste buds and get used to real, whole food, we can no longer accept fake food anymore. It is unfortunate that so many people are so reluctant to break old eating habits, thinking that it will be difficult to make these changes. Once the addiction and nostalgia attachment to high-fat and highly processed foods is broken, our bodies will crave the whole food options.

Fuhrman states in his books that humans have never before had such a vast array of health foods available to them so consistently. Unfortunately, some of us are not yet ready to take advantage of this situation. Instead, the majority of people choose to eat highly processed foods, full of artificial flavors, colorants, and additives.

> It's not that lifestyle interventions don't work—it's just that modest changes are not enough. A slightly lower fat version of the standard American diet cannot complete the demanding task of reversing diabetes. Only radical changes will produce radical results—a radical lifestyle change to a natural, high-nutrient, vegetable-based (nutritarian) eating style, plus frequent exercise. (Joel Fuhrman 2012)

The above statement explains a huge problem. People are induced to think that moderation is the key. However, only radical changes in our diet will produce results that are noticeable. I am one of the thousands who have proved it. It is necessary to eliminate all animal products and all processed foods to see beneficial health improvement. It is also necessary to add a large variety of vegetables, legumes, and fruits on a daily basis.

There is a plethora of incorrect information, spread by the media and marketing industries, clogging websites and TV and radio shows every day. Most of that information comes from corporations that are eager to sell their products. Because of commercial interest, they have created an idyllic image of what it takes to achieve a desired state of health and happiness. Of course, they would have us believe that it is the consumption of their products that is the key. That idea feeds our subconscious minds and induces us to consume addictive products to get us hooked on unhealthy foods.

I have many friends who work in the health industry. It always amazes me how their minds are set on old beliefs that have already been proven inaccurate by serious scientific research.

One of the first things I hear, especially among the older generation, is that animal food is our primary source of protein, calcium, and vitamin D. We all grew up hearing such information. People tell me they drink milk to avoid osteoporosis. People tell me they drink orange juice because it contains vitamin C. People tell me they eat meat and cheese because of their need for protein. While some of these suppositions are true, the life-threatening, negative effects of these foods is overlooked. Few authors have motivated me to learn more about this than T. Colin Campbell. While involved in the China project, which he writes about in his book *The China Study*, there was a long and serious study on the downside of animal protein, casein found in cow's milk, and other dairy products. His research provides strong evidence that casein contributes to the growth of cancer cells. He goes further to explore the problems arising from a high consumption of an animal-rich diet and its relationship to chronic diseases.

I would recommend to anyone interested in improving their health to read T. Colin Campbell's book. He is a serious researcher who has worked in nutrition for more than forty years. We can read about his findings in any of his books: *The China Study* and *Whole: Rethinking the Science of Nutrition*. I found it easy to implement his recommendations and have observed the beneficial results myself in a very short period of time. In spite of starting his research with the intention of promoting the consumption of milk and dairy, he found that "people who ate the most animal-based foods got the most chronic disease ... People who ate the most plant-based foods were the healthiest and tended to avoid chronic diseases" (T. C. Campbell 2004).

Campbell reveals scientific facts about the harm of eating a standard American diet and presents strong evidence against many of the myths our society still believes in and continues to spread (T. C. Campbell 2013). One such myth is the importance of animal milk in our diet. I, like many of you today, used to believe that milk was essential for my health and for my bones. It makes me furious now, after reading so many studies about this subject, that this statement is so far from the truth.

I had heard in the past that humans are the only mammals that drink milk from other species, but the reason for that was never explained to me. I had no idea of the implications of this harmful information, partially because there weren't enough scientific studies easily available to provide evidence of the effects of cow's milk on humans. Fortunately, we now have access to many studies, and we can finally understand these implications. As Dr. Michael Klaper so brilliantly explains: "A calf drinks milk to evolve from a newborn into a mega-tonne heifer in a short period of time. Cow's milk is a hulk-creating substance" (Klaper 2013). Humans easily become addicted to the consumption of milk and dairy products, partially because our society has an obsession with protein intake. Some people have the impression that if we do not ingest huge amounts of animal protein, our lives are in danger. Look around and calculate the amount of protein and fat an average person consumes on a daily basis. It is insane! Meanwhile the lack of nutrients in this very same person's diet could be enormous. Yet no one seems to worry about it.

High amounts of protein and fat will not compensate for the lack of micronutrients in food. The worst thing about this is that people do not realize that the combination of high amounts of protein and fat plus low quantities of nutrients is, in fact, the true cause of many of their chronic diseases.

We are living in a time when much is being questioned about our diets. We could compare this to the '50s and '60s, when people started to realize that smoking was creating serious health issues; that's when the battle against smoking started. Many studies about the harmful effects of smoking may have been done before the public became aware that tobacco was unhealthy. Even though there are still smokers in our midst, the vast majority of us have been persuaded about the detrimental effects of tobacco and choose to avoid even second-hand smoke. I am convinced that the same thing will happen to choices we make about our food. Hopefully, within forty to fifty years, the majority of people on this planet will be converted to a whole, vegetarian diet, composed mostly of vegetables, fruits, legumes, whole grains, seeds, and nuts, thus reducing the number of epidemic, chronic diseases.

Highly processed food is another huge problem in our diet. If an extra-terrestrial empire wanted to take over Earth and kill all humans, it could not find better weapons of destruction than candy and pop.

Candy is the ultimate weapon against the human race: colorful, innocent-looking, attractive, good smelling, good tasting, highly addictive, acidic, and disease forming. Little by little, candy deteriorates the health of humans until it kills them in a slow, painful way. As if candy wasn't bad enough, we have created other foods that are equally morbid: cakes, ice cream, cookies, doughnuts, and pies that are mainly made of highly processed flours, sugars, artificial flavors, and saturated fats.

We evolved without refined sugar, yet in spite of repeated warnings, what do people continue to do? They continue to consume it in large quantities. Even worse, we give it to our children and even bribe them with it. We underestimate the addictive power of sugar.

Many studies have proven that sugar creates the same addiction dependency as cocaine (Marco Aurelio Camargo da Rosa 2012). This means that we feel pleasure when we eat sugar and so we need to increase the amount we eat each time we consume it to feel the same pleasure. And what a pleasure it is! But the worst part is that we persuade our babies and our children to consume it. Not only are we already addicted to it, but we lure every new generation to become dependent on it as well.

Many parents use candy to blackmail children into eating healthier foods. Unfortunately, that does exactly the opposite of what they are trying to accomplish. I define candies as the devil's perfect weapon to destroy humankind. It looks good, tastes wonderful, and undermines our health little by little, disguising itself inside our organs, increasing inflammation, and deteriorating our well-being.

Refined sugar is in almost everything we consume: pop, juice, cake, cookies, sauce, canned food, frozen food, and on and on. I am sure you all know it, so my question to you is this: When are you going to make the decision to finally cut it out of your life?

Yes, there is sugar in fruits ... and vegetables too ... but when sugar comes packed in a fruit or vegetable, it comes with all the other nutrients our bodies need in order to absorb and process this sugar content in a healthy way. It just isn't the same thing.

A plant-based diet is also very helpful to people with coronary disease. In fact, Dr. Caldwell Esselstyn Jr. has a long history of treating his patients with diet and helping them reverse coronary diseases. You can read his concepts and reasoning in his book *Prevent and Reverse Heart Disease*. There are scientific explanations of the damage animal foods create in our bodies. I strongly suggest that you read this author if you decide to explore this topic further.

Chapter 8

Some People Turn a Blind Eye

The future depends on what we do in the present.
—Gandhi

A friend of ours has type 2 diabetes. One day I was talking with his wife when she found out that I had reversed my diabetes. She asked me what I had done, so I gave her a brief explanation of my diet and offered her Dr. Fuhrman's book so she could take a peek. She accepted it and took it home. A couple of weeks later, she told me that it was a very interesting reading but that her husband's diabetes was well under control with medication and the dietary changes would be too hard to endure. I said okay, and that was it. It is not up to me to judge or decide whether someone should or should not change their diet, but I feel an obligation to inform others that there are options available to them.

I know about and have experienced this fantastic way of eating, which people can easily adopt and become, if not completely healthy, much healthier. I feel it is my duty to share it. However, the motivation for change has to come from within. No one can do it for someone else. Even with my loved ones, all I can do is to share my experience and knowledge. Some of my loved ones have seen the difference in my life, and this has convinced them to change their diet as well.

In general, when people are in their twenties, their bodies can take much more abuse. For that reason, it might be difficult for young people to see the damage a standard diet creates. However, a healthy, whole foods, plant-based diet will pay off in the long term.

I want to stress here that a plant-based diet, vegetarian or vegan, is not necessarily healthy in itself. It is imperative to consume a wide variety of whole foods to make a diet healthful. There are highly processed plant foods that are harmful.

I am not suggesting here that we have to eat only vegetables; however, strong evidence has been presented in studies that indicate that a plant-based, whole foods diet is the best for humans. I would like people to think about the content of their daily meals. Most people I observe have a slice of tomato and a lettuce leaf in their burgers or they eat a caesar salad and think they have consumed enough vegetables. I personally like Dr. Fuhrman's suggestion that we should aim to eat at least one pound of raw and one pound of cooked vegetables per day. This has become my rule of thumb.

Vegetables to be consumed in high amounts are all varieties of leafy greens, such as spinach, lettuce, kale, collards, watercress, cabbages, and broccoli, as well as carrots, cauliflower, mushrooms (raw or dried), bell peppers, tomatoes, and so on. Also include fruits, such as berries, grapes, melons, plums, oranges, cherries, and apples, as well as legumes, such as beans, lentils, and all other varieties, plus seeds or nuts. We can still incorporate foods made from whole grains as well.

When I started thinking this way, I discovered a huge amount of food I could rely on. I realized that I would never feel deprived of flavor. It is true that during the first few weeks of my diet change, I did not like the taste of most vegetables. I had to force myself to eat them. I did this because I understood that my quality of life now and later in life would be much better by simply eating plant-based, whole foods rather than starting with medications. Some people prefer the medications since they think they will not need to change anything else. I foresaw a glimpse of my future at the moment when my doctor offered medications: I saw my body deteriorating to the point where I would need a wheelchair and I would still be required to change my diet to include fake, tasteless food that did not resemble what I was used to eating. So my decision was to take the other option. I adopted this diet consisting of high amounts of vegetables. Luckily, I became in control of my own body. The more I implemented this diet, the better I felt. I had it in the back of my head that if this change didn't work, I could always go back to my doctor and start with the medications at a later date. Fortunately, my experiment worked well, and at present, I haven't needed to go back to my doctor and ask for medications.

I have already encouraged other people to make the same decision I did. My wish is that you are the next one. When we get together, we all question the reasons why other people are so reluctant to change the way they eat. There seems to exist a social acceptance that if one does not eat the regular menu offered by the big chain restaurants, one will be deprived. This is so far from the truth!

When I have the opportunity to observe the way people order food in a restaurant or cook at home, I see that they always eat more or less the same food. It seems people are rarely willing to try different food options because they are afraid they will not like new flavors. But here is where it gets interesting: when you make the leap into the world of a vegetable-based diet and make the decision to open your palate to the unknown, there are many nice surprises that await you!

Vegetarian/vegan cuisine has improved so much over the last few years that it is amazing what has been accomplished in terms of good taste. Once you clean out all the toxins that are obstructing your palate, you will find that it is the vegetables, fruits, herbs, and spices that bring flavor to your plate. You will find that you will develop little patience for modified foods anymore. My palate began to distinguish fake versus whole foods very easily. My wish is that you will reach this stage too.

I keep coming across these campaigns for fighting cancer, finding a cure for diabetes, and so forth, and I wonder what is it that people want? There is a cure for most diseases, including cancer, diabetes, high blood pressure, heart problems, and many other chronic illnesses. Eat your vegetables!

Sadly, some people do not want to go through an often lengthy process; they want to believe that a magic pill will allow them to continue abusing their bodies and not take responsibility for a legitimate cure. It is confusing to me that health departments allow the prescribing of so much medication and require so little from family doctors to act in the prevention of their patients' diseases.

I do not have a background in health sciences; however, with some research, I was able to find out what I needed to do to turn my body away from the destructive direction it was heading. I ask myself, "Why is this natural way of eating not widely promoted in our society, especially by governments and health practitioners?"

I know, everyone talks about the multimillion-dollar pharmaceutical companies that would be losing millions of dollars if people did not depend on their products. But how does our government profit from this? Corporate taxes? Am I being naive or is there something going on that we all know about yet nobody is willing to change?

Sometimes people like to feel like the victim. I hear people saying, "I can't eat that because I am diabetic." It sounds to me as though they seek sympathy. "Please feel sorry for me. I want to eat that crappy, sweet cake, and I can't without taking an insulin needle." Really?

Some people like the attention they get when they are in their doctors' offices or in hospitals waiting for treatment or surgery. A dear person in my family is going through this problem as I write. He used to eat tons of meat, potatoes, butter, cheese, milk, bread, and sweets, in addition to drinking beer and other liquor. When my husband and I made the switch to a whole foods plant-based diet, he saw the benefits we achieved, yet he told us that he would never be able to eat only "grass." Well, a year and a half later, he was waiting for coronary surgery. What surprises me is that he seems okay with it. However, I am sure he didn't realize that he would have to change his diet after the surgery. His energy will never be the same. This person is three years younger than I am, and I could have been in a very similar situation if I had not made changes in my life. It was difficult to change, but is surgery less difficult? It only seems this way because it is faster and everyone around is sympathetic.

Thus, I think instead of trashing the idea of eating a whole foods, plant-based diet and increasing the amount of vegetables we eat, we should embrace it and start making it sound appealing and a worthy cause. Then many more people would join this movement, and "eat for a cure" would help prevent many of us from having major surgery, chemotherapy, and many other traumatic treatments.

Of course, the medical, pharmaceutical, and food industries will likely oppose any movement that affects their source of revenue. But it would be very beneficial for the rest of us.

There are so many alternatives for healthful eating out there that it becomes difficult to make up our minds. So I hope to help you analyze what is most important and make it easier for you to pay attention to your own needs.

I have tried numerous diets throughout my life. The only one I was able to maintain was this unprocessed vegan diet with no added sugar, oil, or salt. Sometimes, when I am at social functions, people still try to convince me that what they are eating is good for me. I have to stick to my views, knowing the truth about the benefits of my choice. Since I have started this diet, I not only lost eighty-nine pounds without regaining it, but, more important, I was able to get back to normal in all my body functions. My blood tests show normal ranges whereas before my glucose was extremely high, my cholesterol was high, and many other functions were out of whack.

Every time I want to eat something outside of my diet, I have to remind myself of my goal, and that goal continues to be to stay well for as long as I can, without depending on medication or any other medical treatment.

I understand that it seems to be too thought-provoking to think about adopting a whole foods plant-based diet when one is still at a young age, but the ideal for our health would be to create a habit of eating for life as early as possible. Changes later in life are possible and beneficial but much more complex to implement.

Our society has perfected a system of increasing the taste of foods artificially in order to give us the highest possible pleasure when eating. This is because we live in a society that suppresses many of our natural ways to release anxiety and feel pleasure. Eating has become the easiest way to achieve pleasure, and for this reason, much emphasis is put into enhancing flavors. Such perfection has its price, and the price we pay is a detriment to the quality of what we eat.

Our bodies are so perfectly designed that they have built-in abilities to detox and heal themselves whenever they are attacked. We all have these instincts, and they work perfectly if we give them the ideal conditions in which to do so.

In the past century, people have decided that, because of their inventions, they are smarter than nature, and they keep insisting on inventing better ways for our bodies to heal. Yet nature does it perfectly, and we already know that, but we keep insisting on stuffing ourselves with manipulated, processed, "quality" food and then trying to find a way around it by ingesting supplements or more of the same foods.

Unfortunately, the food industry is feeding both the pharmaceutical industry and the medical system. The health system we have in practice in the West at the moment treats symptoms instead of the causes of our diseases. When we rely on symptom relief, we immediately forget that there is a cause that has to be addressed. Symptoms are one of the tools our body uses to let us know that there is something wrong with us. We should pay careful attention and address that problem. One way of doing so is by noticing what is happening in our bodies, observing what we are consuming, getting rid of the bad foods or bad habits, and getting back into a lifestyle with a more nourishing diet.

Some people will rely on medical advice and pharmaceutical drugs and will suppress their symptoms and continue to ingest very low-quality food in large amounts. Such behavior quite often contributes to the growth of the ailment and to the continuous use of pharmaceutical drugs.

Chapter 9

Implementing a New Diet

The time will come when men such as I will look upon the murder of animals as they now look upon the murder of men.
—Leonardo Da Vinci

O ver the span of two years, since adopting the whole foods, plant-based diet, I have had the opportunity to host family and friends in my house for periods of a month or two. Everyone who comes for a visit is exposed to the benefits of this diet and has the opportunity to find out how it works and how easy and tasty it is to implement. It is very interesting to observe that when they arrive in my house, they are curious but still have many prejudices against eating mostly vegetables and fruits. First, they think there is not enough protein; second, they think it will be boring and lacking in flavor.

I always offer them the freedom to eat the way they want and to prepare their own food if they wish. Some of them do so at the beginning, but as time goes by, and they see everyone in the family having so much pleasure eating more healthfully, they start eating like us. They agree that the food is delicious and that they do not need to eat the junk they were used to before. So I have taught a few nephews, nieces, and friends to enjoy and appreciate my diet. But what happens after they go back to their regular lives? This is what is interesting. They forget what they have experienced here, and they go back to their regular old unhealthful habits. I think this happens because of the influence of the people around them, which makes it too difficult, in their minds, to continue with new habits. When there is no one else to share and support the alternative lifestyle, it tends to dissolve.

It is very important to bring awareness to people, but we also have to go beyond; we have to help people implement healthy diets as part of their regular daily routines.

Our society has created a pleasure-eating trap where our biggest goal is to eat as much as possible of the foods we enjoy, without thinking of the consequences. How are we going to address such a problem?

We might have to reinvent our restaurants and start having more and more access to whole, plant-based foods on a daily basis. Whole foods satisfy our hunger for a longer period of time. The availability of vegetarian food has improved in the past decade, but we are still far away from an ideal situation. The day will come when restaurant owners and chefs will find out that it is simpler and costless to provide a delicious healthful meal to their clients. It will be possible to increase their profits, and that might be a strong incentive to bring plant-based whole foods to the public.

People who still want animal foods in their diet could continue to eat these in moderate amounts, as villagers in the West have done in past centuries (Montignac n.d.). It is interesting to find out what people ate in the past and the assumptions we make around their diet and lifestyle. There are many studies suggesting that people ate animal products only occasionally because it was difficult to hunt and have access to these products. Animal food was more common when there was a shortage of vegetables. Yet some of us are under the impression that meat was widely available to everyone, every day in primitive societies (Warinner 2014). Vegetables, fruits, and legumes were restricted to certain places in the world due to climate fluctuation; however, we have resolved these shortages, at least for the most developed countries. There is an abundant selection of vegetables, fruits, legumes, grains, seeds, and nuts available on a daily basis. Never before have we been so fortunate in the variety of our food selection.

Another very complicated problem we have today is the complexity of our dishes. It seems very important to have a large combination of ingredients in our recipes, while, from my point of view, a daily diet should be simple. Cooks and chefs have been experimenting with recipes based on animal food and highly processed ingredients for many years. It is very easy to understand that our taste buds crave meats, sweets, oil, and salt while we become very addicted to them. Not only do we use too many addictive ingredients in our dishes, but we are also in the habit of overcooking plants. It is easy to find places where vegetables are mushy and tasteless. The time has arrived where experiments in the kitchen should be focused on foods as they come from nature.

Here is my suggestion for introducing a plant-based diet: Cook simply, one vegetable at a time. Add only seasonings that you like. Cook lightly, using whatever method you prefer. The healthiest ways to eat vegetables are raw, steamed, cooked in water, baked, water-sautéed, grilled, and, lastly, fried.

Getting Started

Start by ridding your house of all unhealthy foods that you no longer intend to eat. Go to the supermarket and stock up on plenty of fresh and frozen fruits and vegetables.

Fill up on large quantities of high-nutrient, low-calorie foods first and then eat the higher calorie foods. Always eat high-nutrient foods before lower nutrient ones.

Try to use a variety of vegetables every day since this will bring more complete nutrients and vitamins to your body.

It is easy to lose weight and reverse chronic diet-related diseases following this guideline without the need to count calories or add supplements.

Suggested Shopping List

Whole Grains

amaranth

brown rice

buckwheat

farro

millet

oats

quinoa

teff

whole wheat flour

wild rice

Fruits

apples

avocados

bananas

blueberries (fresh and frozen)

dates

lemons juice or fresh lemons for
    juicing

lemons

limes

mandarin oranges

oranges

papaya

peaches

pears

pineapple

raspberries (fresh and frozen)

strawberries (fresh and frozen)

Vegetables

baby corn (fresh or canned)

baby spinach (fresh)

bean sprouts

bell peppers (green/red/yellow)

broccoli florets

cabbage green

carrots

celery

collard greens

corn on the cob

eggplants

garlic (chopped)

green beans (fresh)

kale

lettuce (fresh, any type)

mushrooms (fresh, any type)

onions (any type)

pickle-sized cucumbers

potatoes (any type)

radishes

romaine lettuce

snow peas

spaghetti squash

spinach (fresh)

swiss chard (fresh, red or white)

tomatoes (fresh or canned)

Beans

any canned beans, no salt added

black beans

chickpeas

garbanzo beans (dried or canned)

green split peas (dried)

lentils (red or brown)

red beans

tofu, extra firm

white beans

Nuts and Seeds

almonds (raw)

cashew butter

cashew nuts (raw)

flaxseed

pumpkin seeds (raw)

sesame seeds (raw)

sunflower seeds (raw)

walnuts (raw)

Seasonings

balsamic vinegar

basil

Bragg Liquid Aminos

caraway seeds

cilantro

cinnamon

coriander ground

cumin seeds

curry powder

date sugar

dill

dried basil

fresh garlic

garlic powder

gingerroot

ground mustard

minced onion flakes

mustard, salt-free

onion powder

paprika

parsley (dried)

red pepper flakes

turmeric

vanilla extract

Chapter 10

Recipes

The ideal human diet looks like this: Consume plant-based foods in forms as close to their natural state as possible ("whole" foods). Eat a variety of vegetables, fruits, raw nuts and seeds, beans and legumes, and whole grains. Avoid heavily processed foods and animal products. Stay away from added salt, oil, and sugar. Aim to get 80 percent of your calories from carbohydrates, 10 percent from fat, and 10 percent from protein.
—T. Colin Campbell

R ecipes I normally use in my kitchen will be described below. Some of them are my own creation; others are someone else's creation. Quite often I have modified original recipes to adapt to my particular taste. I will be referencing the sources when they are not my creation.

I believe that delicious recipes should be freely exchanged mainly because we are so inexperienced in healthy eating habits that the more we share, the more we improve each other's health. I also believe that the more people eat plant-based foods, the more they will like and want them. It is equally important to learn to eat when we are hungry and not just because we want to fit into the patterns of society.

Chefs strive to make their dishes appealing to their customers. Each time one of us asks for vegan foods, chefs will take up the challenge and create a dish with vegan characteristics. Good chefs take pride in creating dishes that are in demand from their customers. In conclusion, if we start demanding simpler and healthier dishes, eventually we will have a society that eats well, preventing a great number of diseases. Today more than ever, it is imperative that we create a conscious demand for large quantities of vegetables on a daily basis.

The recipes I propose are mostly a simple combination of whole, vegetarian ingredients. Substitutions can be readily made, if you prefer. There is no secret to these recipes; the skill level to prepare most of my recipes is basic.

Smoothies and Juices

To make smoothies, a blender (the higher the power, the better) is required for ease of preparation. Having said that, by using a simple technique of combining the greens with the liquid first and then adding the other ingredients, you can get good results with a regular blender. I find smoothies also taste better when I use frozen fruits. The nice thing about smoothies is that they help me fill up on greens and fiber.

Juices are delicious too, but they exclude a large part of the food, so they are not really whole foods. I use them as a treat.

Remember to always present your smoothies and juices in beautiful glassware because it gives us the visual satisfaction that influences our palate.

1. Melon Avocado Smoothie

Prep Time: 5 minutes   Yield: 1 serving

Ingredients

1 cup baby spinach leaves
1 cup frozen melon, diced
1/4 avocado, diced
1/2 lime, juiced

2 pitted dates
1 tablespoon chia seed
1 cup of water

Directions

In a regular blender, liquefy green leaves and liquids first.
Add remaining ingredients and blend about 2 minutes, until very smooth.
Serve in a beautiful crystal glass, and enjoy.

2. Berry Banana Smoothie

Prep Time: 5 minutes   Yield: 1 serving

Ingredients
1 cup baby spinach leaves   1/2 cup frozen raspberries
1 cup frozen blueberries   1 tablespoon flaxseeds
1/2 banana   1 cup water

Directions
In a regular blender, liquefy green leaves and liquids first.
Add remaining ingredients and blend about 2 minutes, until very smooth.
Serve in a beautiful crystal glass, and enjoy.

3. Avocado Pineapple Smoothie

Prep Time: 5 minutes   Yield: 1 serving

Ingredients
1 cup baby spinach leaves   2 pitted dates
1 cup frozen pineapple   1 tablespoon pecans
1/2 cup pineapple juice   1 cup of water
1 avocado

Directions
In a regular blender, liquefy green leaves and liquids first.
Add remaining ingredients and blend about 2 minutes, until very smooth.
Serve in a beautiful crystal glass, and enjoy.

4. Chocolate Cherry Smoothie (Dr. Fuhrman n.d.)

Prep Time: 6 minutes   Yield: 2 servings

Ingredients

1 cup baby spinach
1 cup romaine lettuce
1/2 cup unsweetened soy, hemp, or almond milk
1/2 cup pomegranate juice or cherry juice

1 tablespoon cocoa powder
1 cup frozen cherries
1 ripe banana
1 cup frozen blueberries
1/2 teaspoon vanilla extract
2 tablespoon ground flaxseeds

Directions

In a regular blender, liquefy green leaves and liquids first.
Add remaining ingredients and blend about 2 minutes, until very smooth.
Serve in a beautiful crystal glass, and enjoy.

5. Guava Papaya Smoothie

Prep Time: 5 minutes   Yield: 1 serving

Ingredients

1 cup iceberg lettuce
1/2 cup swiss chard
1/2 lime, juiced
1 guava

1/2 papaya
1 tablespoon sunflower seeds
1 cup coconut water

Directions

In a regular blender, liquefy green leaves and liquids first.
Add remaining ingredients and blend about 2 minutes, until very smooth.
Serve in a beautiful crystal glass, and enjoy.

6. Raspberry Cocoa Smoothie

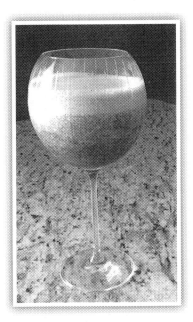

Prep Time: 5 minutes
Yield: 1 serving

Ingredients
1 cup collard greens, stems removed
1 cup frozen raspberries
1/2 lime, juiced
1 banana
1 tablespoon raw cocoa
2 pitted dates
1 teaspoon vanilla extract
1 cup of water

Directions
In a regular blender, liquefy green leaves and liquids first.
Add remaining ingredients and blend about 2 minutes, until very smooth.
Serve in a beautiful crystal glass, and enjoy.

7. Red Orange Smoothie

Prep Time: 5 minutes   Yield: 1 serving

Ingredients
1/2 cup swiss chard
1/2 cup beet greens
1 cup frozen mango cubes
1/2 papaya
1 cup pineapple cubes

1 teaspoon vanilla extract
2 pitted dates
1 tablespoon flaxseed
1 cup water

Directions
In a regular blender, liquefy green leaves and liquids first.
Add remaining ingredients and blend about 2 minutes, until very smooth.
Serve in a beautiful crystal glass, and enjoy.

8. Kiwi Melon Smoothie

Prep Time: 5 minutes   Yield: 1 serving

Ingredients
1 cup almond milk

1 cup kale, stems removed

1 cup swiss chard

1 cup frozen honeydew melon

1 cup kiwi

1/4 apple

1 teaspoon stevia powder

1 tablespoon sesame seed

Directions
In a regular blender, liquefy green leaves and liquids first.

Add remaining ingredients and blend about 2 minutes, until very smooth.

Serve in a beautiful crystal glass, and enjoy.

Juices

I love juices because they make it easy to get an abundance of vitamins right into our bloodstream. When I exercise and drink a beet juice right after, I can feel the rush of the vitamins in my body. What a refreshing sensation! Another great time for me to drink a vegetable juice is after dinner when people normally sip a glass of wine. I feel empowered by the amount of nutrients in my body, and I feel them working overnight. Whatever time you decide to enjoy your vegetable juice is a good time, but don't drink it as a replacement for your veggies. Consider it a treat.

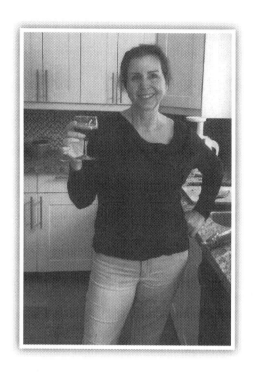

1. **Kicking Kale Juice** (Colins 2015)

Prep Time: 10 minutes   Yield: 1 serving

Ingredients
2 celery stalks

1 lemon, peeled

2 green apples

4 leaves kale

1/8 teaspoon grated ginger

Directions
Process all ingredients in your juicer.

You can vary the amount of kick the juice has by adding more ginger.

Serve in a wineglass.

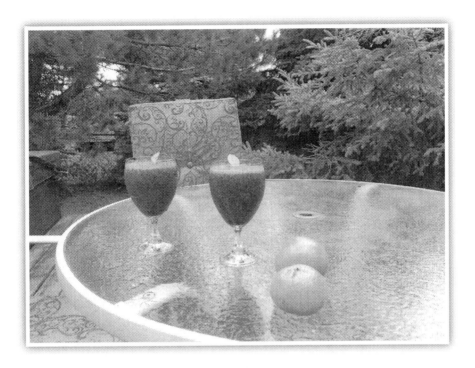

2. Divine Fresh Wine

Prep Time: 10 minutes   Yield: 2 servings

Ingredients

2 beets

1 lemon, peeled

2 carrots

1 apple

2 inches gingerroot

Directions

Process all ingredients in your juicer.

Serve in a wineglass.

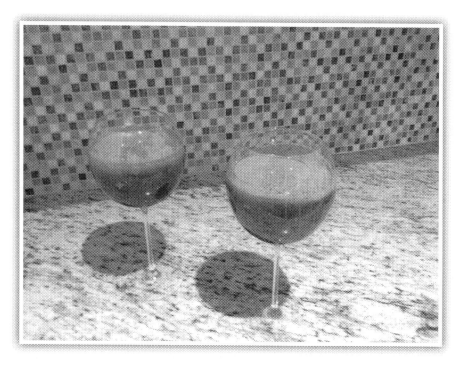

3. Not Wine

Prep Time: 10 minutes   Yield: 2 servings

Ingredients

2 beets

1 lemon, peeled

2 carrots

1 apple

4 leaves kale

Directions

Process all ingredients in your juicer.

Serve in a wineglass.

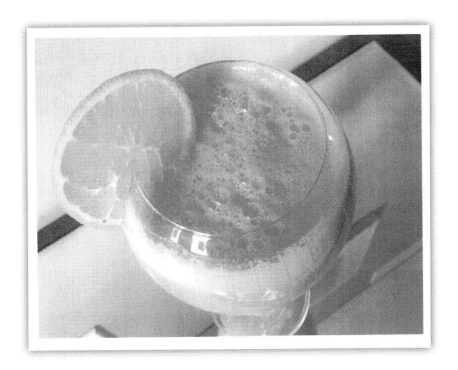

4. Vital Beta C

Prep Time: 10 minutes   Yield: 2 servings

Ingredients
3 oranges, peeled
1 cup pineapple
1 large sweet potato

Directions
Process all ingredients to your juicer.
Serve in a wineglass.

5. Swiss Combination

Prep Time: 10 minutes   Yield: 2 servings

Ingredients
1 cucumber   1/2 cup of pineapple
1 apple   4 kale leaves
1 lemon, peeled   3 swiss chard leaves

Directions
Process all ingredients to your juicer.
Serve in a wineglass.

6. Mellow Apple

Prep Time: 10 minutes   Yield: 2 servings

Ingredients
2 cups watermelon   1/2 lemon, peeled
2 apples   4 kale leaves

Directions
Process all ingredients to your juicer.
Serve in a wineglass.

7. Blood Orange and Apple

Prep Time: 10 minutes   Yield: 2 servings

Ingredients

1 cucumber

3 celery stalks

3 swiss chard leaves

1 bell pepper

1 beet

1 apple

1 blood orange, peeled

Directions

Process all ingredients to your juicer.

Serve in a wineglass.

Salads

Salad should be the main dish of the meal. I discovered that salads are very important because they bring an abundance of nutrients and fiber to our bodies. Normally, when we make our salads at home, we just pick and choose among the vegetables that we have in the fridge, and we don't use any dressing other than lime, lemon, or pineapple juice. They taste amazing! The addition of fruits and seeds brings a dance of flavor that is lacking in regular salads.

My personal guideline is to use two or three green, leafy vegetables, one or two varieties of seeds or nuts, two or three fruits, as well as one red and one yellow vegetable. Below you will find a couple of suggestions for salads that we have experimented with and enjoyed. The combinations are limitless, and I can say that very rarely do we make the same recipe. This, by itself, gives us a diversity of nutrients, which is ideal. So explore my recipes and don't be afraid to modify them and create your own.

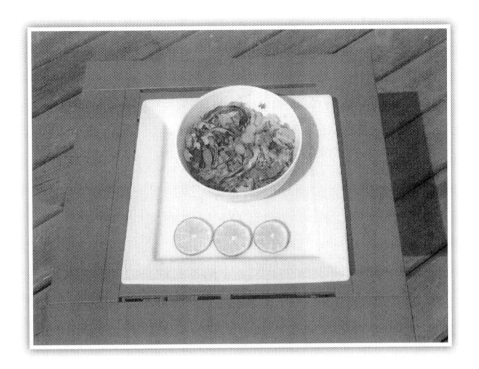

1. Daily Green Salad

Prep Time: 20 minutes   Yield: 3 servings

Ingredients

1 bunch kale, chopped
1 head romaine lettuce, roughly
   chopped
1 cup red cabbage, chopped
2 carrots, sliced

1 red onion, chopped
1 clove garlic, minced
1/2 lime, juiced
3 tablespoons pumpkin seeds
1/4 cup of raw almonds

Directions

Mix leafy vegetables in a bowl.
Stir in lime juice, almonds, and pumpkin seeds.
Add remaining ingredients, and mix well.

2. Arugula Romaine Salad

Prep Time: 20 minutes   Yield: 3 servings

Ingredients
1/4 pound arugula
1 heart of romaine lettuce
8 radishes, sliced
3 leek stalks, sliced

1 apple, diced
1/2 lemon, juiced
3 tablespoons raw sunflower
    seeds

Directions
Mix leafy vegetables in a bowl.
Stir in lime juice and sunflower seeds.
Add remaining ingredients, and mix well.

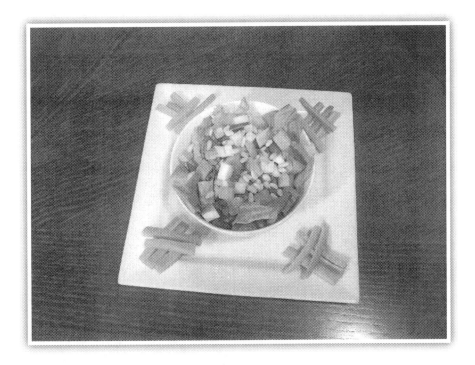

3. Boston Romaine Salad

Prep Time: 20 minutes   Yield: 3 servings

Ingredients

1 head boston lettuce
1 heart romaine lettuce
1 cup green beans
1 carrot, diced

1 apple, diced
1/2 lime, juiced
1 cup pine nuts

Directions

Mix leafy vegetables in a bowl.
Stir in lime juice and pine nuts.
Add remaining ingredients, and mix well.

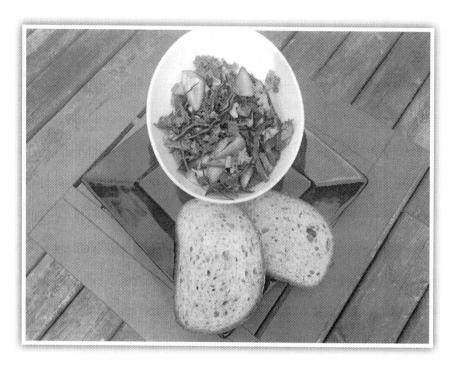

4. Red and Green Salad

Prep Time: 20 minutes   Yield: 3 servings

Ingredients

6 collard green leaves, with stems
1 bunch boston lettuce
2 roma tomatoes, diced
2 carrots, diced

2 cups strawberry, sliced
1/2 lemon, juiced
1/4 cup raw almonds

Directions

Mix leafy vegetables in a bowl.
Stir in lemon juice and almonds.
Add remaining ingredients, and mix well.

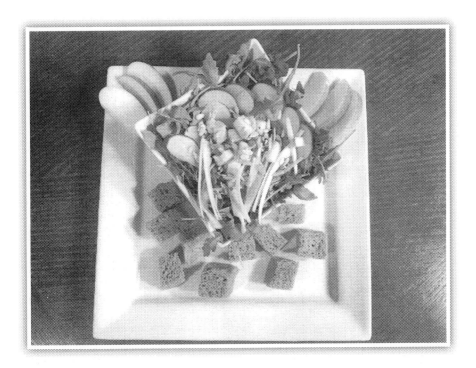

5. Kale Arugula Salad

Prep Time: 20 minutes   Yield: 3 servings

Ingredients
1 bunch kale, chopped
2 cups arugula leaves
1 cup radish, finely sliced
3 leek stalks, sliced

1 cup raspberries
1/2 lemon, juiced
1/2 cup chia seeds

Directions
Mix leafy vegetables in a bowl.
Stir in lime juice and chia seeds.
Add remaining ingredients, and mix well.

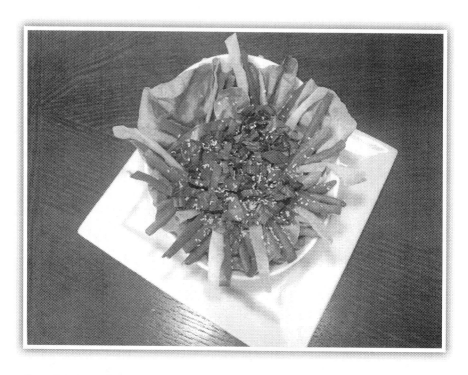

6. Boston Chard Salad

Prep Time: 20 minutes   Yield: 3 servings

Ingredients

5 leaves swiss chard, finely
   chopped
1 bunch boston lettuce, chopped
1 cup cooked or canned green
   beans

1 red bell pepper, cut into strips
1 mango, cut into strips
1/2 lime, juiced
1/2 cup sesame seeds, lightly
   toasted

Directions

Mix leafy vegetables in a bowl.
Stir in lime juice and sesame seeds.
Add remaining ingredients, and mix well.

7. Red "Cash" Salad

Prep Time: 20 minutes   Yield: 3 servings

Ingredients

1 bunch kale, chopped
1 cup red cabbage, chopped
1 beet, diced
1 large red onion, diced

1 cup strawberry, sliced
1/2 lime, juiced
1/4 cup of raw cashews

Directions

Mix leafy vegetables in a bowl.
Stir in lime juice and cashews.
Add remaining ingredients, and mix well.

8. Amazing Vegan Cheese Sauce (to be used as salad dressing) (Anthony 2015)

Prep Time: 40 minutes   Yield: 4 servings

Ingredients

3 medium potatoes, chopped
7 medium carrots, chopped
1/2 cup water, used to boil
    potatoes
1/4 cup plus 2 tablespoons
    nutritional yeast

1–2 tablespoons lemon juice
1 teaspoon salt
1/2 teaspoon onion powder
1/2 teaspoon garlic powder
1/2 teaspoon brown mustard
1/8 tablespoon turmeric

Directions

Peel potatoes and carrots, if desired.
Cut them into small cubes, and boil for 10 minutes.
Let rest for 5 minutes.
Drain vegetables, and transfer to blender.
Add 1/2 cup potato water, and pulse to mix.
Add remaining ingredients; blend until smooth and creamy.

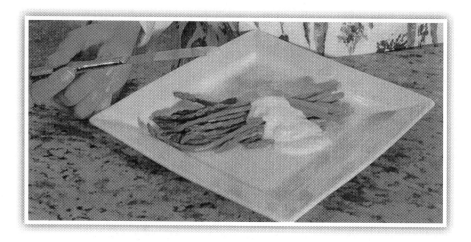

9. Asparagus with Vegan Hollandaise
(Vegetarian Times 2011)

Prep Time: 30 minutes   Yield: 3 servings

Classic hollandaise sauce is mostly egg yolks and butter (with a few seasonings thrown in), making it one of the worst offenders for saturated fat. Steamed silken tofu gives you the same creamy consistency, and there is no worry about the sauce curdling or turning. This version can be made ahead and reheated by stirring over low heat just until warm.

Ingredients

1/2 cup silken tofu
2 tablespoons lemon juice
1 tablespoon nutritional yeast
1/2 teaspoon salt

1/8 tablespoon cayenne pepper
1/8 tablespoon turmeric
2 tablespoons corn oil
2 pounds asparagus, trimmed

Directions

Heat tofu in water bath for 45 seconds, or until warm.
Add lemon juice, nutritional yeast, salt, cayenne, and turmeric to a food processor, add warm tofu, and purée until smooth.
With food processor running, add oil in steady stream to finish sauce.
Steam asparagus for 2 minutes, or until crisp-tender.
Drain and serve with sauce.

10. Broccoli and Chickpea Salad (Dr. Fuhrman n.d.)

Prep Time: 15 minutes   Yield: 4 servings

Ingredients

For the Salad
6 cups broccoli, cut into small florets
1 can chickpeas, no salt added, drained
1/4 cup red onion, chopped
1 1/2 cups cherry tomatoes, halved
1/4 cup pine nuts or walnuts, toasted

For the Dressing
1/4 cup fresh lemon juice
1/2 cup water
1/4 cup walnuts
1/4 cup dates, chopped
1 teaspoon dijon mustard
1 clove garlic

Directions
Steam broccoli until just tender, 5–7 minutes.
Once cool, combine with chickpeas, onion, cherry tomatoes, and nuts.
Blend dressing ingredients in a high-powered blender.
Toss salad with desired amount of dressing.
Leftover dressing may be reserved for another use.

11. Four Bean Salad

Prep: 15 minutes   Yield: 3 servings

Ingredients
1 can dark kidney beans, rinsed and drained
1 can cannellini beans, rinsed and drained
1 can black beans, rinsed and drained
1 can garbanzo beans, rinsed and drained
2 cups corn, fresh or frozen
1 large red bell pepper, diced
1/2 cup red onion, finely chopped
1/4 cup vinegar
juice of 1 lemon
2 teaspoons ground cumin
1 teaspoon ground coriander
1/8 tablespoon cayenne pepper

Directions
Place all beans in a large bowl.
Add bell pepper, onion, and corn.
Mix remaining ingredients together, and pour over the salad.
Toss gently to mix.

12. **Kale Fattoush** (Center for Nutrition Studies 2015)

Prep Time: 20 minutes   Yield: 4 servings

Ingredients

7 ounces kale

2 shallots

10 small tomatoes

8 red-skinned radishes

1 zucchini, spiralized

5 sprigs fresh mint, chopped

5 sprigs fresh parsley, chopped

2 wholemeal pita or flatbreads

For the Dressing

juice of 1/2 lemon

1 clove garlic

3 teaspoons olive oil

2 teaspoons apple cider vinegar

1 teaspoon sumac

1/4 teaspoon salt (optional)

1/4 teaspoon black pepper

Directions

Remove stems, and tear kale leaves into bite-size pieces.

Place kale in a large bowl.

Combine all dressing ingredients in a separate bowl, and mix.

Pour dressing over the kale, and massage the leaves until they are bright green and tender.

Slice shallots thinly, and add to the kale; allow the mixture to marinate.

Cut tomatoes in half.

Slice the radishes into slivers.

Chop the leaves of the mint and parsley.

Add tomatoes, radishes, zucchini, mint, and parsley to the kale.

Toast the bread, cut into little squares, and stir in.

13. Mango-Lime Salad (*To Lower Cholesterol Naturally* 2011)

Prep Time: 10 minutes   Yield: 2 servings

Ingredients

1 mango, peeled and diced

1/2 red onion, diced (add more or less, to taste)

1 can cannellini beans, drained and rinsed

1/2 cup cilantro (add more to taste)

juice or zest of lemon

baby lettuce or arugula

Directions

Combine all ingredients.

Serve on a bed of greens.

14. Chickpea Zucchini Salad

Prep Time: 20 minutes   Yield: 3 servings

Ingredients

3 small zucchinis

1 can chickpeas, rinsed and drained

1/2 cup red onion, chopped

1/2 large red bell pepper

2 cloves garlic, minced

2 tablespoons lemon juice

2 tablespoons white balsamic or white wine vinegar

1/2 teaspoon black pepper

salt, to taste (optional)

fresh herbs (such as mint, basil, or oregano) to taste

Directions

Cut zucchinis in half, and slice.

Cut bell pepper into fine, long slices.

Combine all ingredients in a bowl.

Add seasonings and fresh herbs.

15. MiracleNaise: Soy-Free, Vegan Mayo
(Voisin, *Fat Free Vegan Kitchen* 2014)

Prep Time: 6 minutes　　　Yield: 200 milliliters

Ingredients
1 can artichoke quarters, drained well
1/4 cup raw cashews soaked in water for a few hours, drained
2 tablespoon water
1 teaspoon stone-ground mustard
1/8 teaspoon xanthan gum, to thicken (optional)
salt and lemon juice (optional)

Directions
Place all ingredients into a high-speed blender and process until completely smooth.
Taste and, if necessary, add salt and a few drops of lemon juice.
Refrigerate and use within 2 weeks.

16. Mixed Greens and Strawberry Salad (Dr. Fuhrman n.d.)

Prep Time: 15 minutes   Yield: 3 servings

Ingredients

For the Salad
1 head romaine lettuce
5 ounces baby spinach
4 cups sliced strawberries, fresh or frozen (defrosted)

For the Dressing
1/4 cup raw cashews or 2 tablespoons raw cashew butter
1/3 cup unsweetened soy or almond milk
1 apple, peeled and cored
2 tablespoons dried currants or raisins

Directions
Place lettuce and spinach leaves on a plate.
Top with strawberries.
Blend all dressing ingredients until smooth.
Drizzle dressing over the greens and berries.

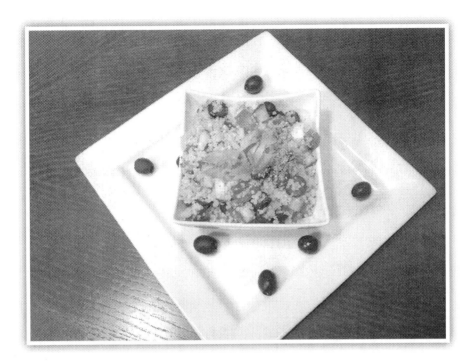

17. Quinoa Salad

Prep Time: 15 minutes   Yield: 4 servings

Ingredients

1 cup previously cooked quinoa
2 celery stalks, sliced
1 cucumber, diced
1 red pepper, diced
6 cherry tomatoes
1/2 cup black olives, sliced

2 tablespoons olive oil
1/2 cup lemon juice
3 tablespoons white vinegar
salt and pepper, to taste
2 tablespoons oregano

Directions

Combine all ingredients together, and mix well.
Enjoy!

18. Red Cabbage Coleslaw (Dr. Fuhrman n.d.)

Prep Time: 20 minutes   Yield: 4 servings

Ingredients
3 cups red cabbage, shredded
1 cup carrots, shredded
1 tablespoon cilantro, chopped
2 tablespoons scallions, sliced
1 tablespoon fruity vinegar
3 tablespoons apricot puree (note below)
1 tablespoon unsalted natural peanut butter
1 teaspoon low-sodium soy sauce
2 teaspoons sesame seeds, lightly toasted

Note: Place 1/4 cup dried apricots in a glass bowl. Add 1/4 cup boiling water. Let stand for 15 minutes or until apricots are soft. Transfer to a food processor, and blend the apricots and water until smooth.

Directions
In a large bowl, combine red cabbage, carrots, cilantro, and scallions. In a small bowl, combine remaining ingredients, and mix until smooth. Add mixture to red cabbage and carrots.

19. Spinach Salad with Curry Dressing
(Center for Nutrition Studies 2015)

Prep Time: 25 minutes   Yield: 3 servings

Ingredients
1 bunch fresh spinach, washed
1/3 cup peanuts
1 tart green apple, diced
2 scallions, thinly sliced, including green tops
1/4 cup raisins
1 tablespoon sesame seeds
3 tablespoons vinegar
3 tablespoons frozen apple juice concentrate
2 teaspoons stone-ground or dijon mustard
1 teaspoon low-sodium soy sauce
1/2 teaspoon curry powder
1/4 teaspoon black pepper

Directions
Spread peanuts and sesame seeds on an oven-proof pan and bake at 375°F for 15 minutes. Let cool.
Combine spinach with apple, scallions, and raisins in a large salad bowl. Add cooled peanuts and sesame seeds.
Whisk vinegar, apple juice concentrate, mustard, soy sauce, curry powder, and black pepper together in a small bowl.
Just before serving, pour over the salad and toss to mix.

Soups

Soups are extremely important in this diet. They not only heat our body during cold times, but they bring us an abundance of nutrients, fiber, and water. I like my soups spicy and hot in temperature. If you don't like them spicy, just ignore the hot spices in the recipe. Another benefit of soups is that you can use the leftovers from another meal and combine them by adding water and other fresh ingredients. This makes a super-easy soup, ready in just minutes. I do this quite often when I have leftover beans or steamed veggies. I prefer to chew my veggies, and I keep them al dente, so I rarely blend my soups, but feel free to blend them if that is more appealing to your palate. For people who are transitioning from a standard diet, soups are very important because they fulfill that desire to eat or snack on something, simply by enjoying a bowl of soup. So go crazy on soups!

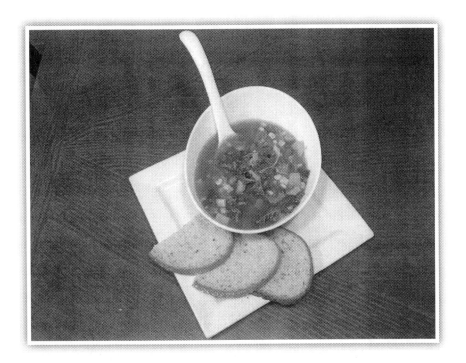

1. Kale Carrot Soup

Prep Time: 25 minutes   Yield: 3 servings

Ingredients

1 onion, diced
3 kale leaves, coarsely chopped
3 carrots, diced
100 grams brussels sprouts, cut in half
2 celery stalks, sliced
1 cup corn kernels
1 tablespoon balsamic vinegar
3 fresh tomatoes, diced
4 cups water
1 tablespoon onion powder
1 tablespoon paprika
1 teaspoon black pepper (optional)

Directions

Water-sauté onions in a pan until softened.

Add carrots, brussels sprouts, and 2 cups of hot water.

Bring to a boil; then reduce heat and simmer for 10 minutes.

Add all other ingredients except kale.

Add remaining 2 cups of water.

Cook at medium heat for another 15 minutes.

Adjust the water if needed.

Stir in kale, and heat until kale is wilted.

Turn off the heat. Serve immediately.

2. Green Spinach Soup

Prep Time: 25 minutes   Yield: 3 servings

Ingredients

1 white onion, diced

2 cups spinach

2 sweet potatoes

100 grams brussels sprouts

1 red onion, diced

1 cup white giant beans

1 cup parsley

3 fresh tomatoes, diced

4 cups water

1 tablespoon onion powder

1 tablespoon curry powder

1 teaspoon black pepper
  (optional)

Directions

Water-sauté white onions in a pan until softened.

Add beans, potatoes, brussels sprouts, and 2 cups of hot water.

Bring to a boil; then reduce heat and simmer for 10 minutes.

Add all other ingredients except spinach.

Add remaining 2 cups of water.

Cook at medium heat for another 15 minutes.

Adjust the water if needed.

Stir in spinach, and heat until spinach is wilted.

Turn off the heat. Serve immediately.

3. Curry Lentils and Collard Greens Soup

Prep Time: 25 minutes   Yield: 3 servings

Ingredients:
1 onion, diced
2 russet potatoes, cubed
2 cups butternut squash, cubed
1 cup green lentils
2 zucchinis, diced
3 collard greens leaves, coarsely sliced
1 tablespoon balsamic vinegar
1 can diced tomatoes
5 cups water
1 tablespoon onion powder
1 tablespoon curry powder
1 teaspoon black pepper (optional)

Directions
Water-sauté onions in a pan until softened.
Add potatoes, butternut squash, lentils, and 3 cups of hot water. Bring to a boil.
Reduce heat, and let it simmer for 10 minutes.
Add all other ingredients except collard greens.
Add remaining 2 cups of water.
Cook at medium heat for another 15 minutes.
Adjust the water if necessary.
Stir in collard greens, and heat until they are wilted.
Turn off heat. Serve immediately.

4. Cabbage Potato Soup

Prep Time: 25 minutes   Yield: 3 servings

Ingredients
1 onion, diced
2 russet potatoes, cubed
1 cup red cabbage, shredded
1 cup green peas
2 celery stalks, sliced
1 cup corn kernels
3 fresh tomatoes, diced
1 tablespoon shoyu
4 cups water
1 tablespoon onion powder
1 tablespoon garlic powder
1 tablespoon paprika
1 teaspoon cayenne pepper (optional)

Directions
Water-sauté onions in a pan until softened.
Add potatoes, cabbage, and 2 cups of hot water; bring to a boil.
Reduce heat, and let it simmer for 10 minutes.
Add all other ingredients.
Add remaining 2 cups of water.
Cook at medium heat for another 15 minutes.
Adjust the water as required.
Turn off the heat. Serve immediately.

5.   White Bean Soup

Prep Time: 60 minutes   Yield: 3 servings

Ingredients

1 cup white giant beans, dry
2 russet potatoes, cubed
2 cups butternut squash, cubed
1 onion, diced
1 cup cabbage, shredded
1 cup green beans, lozenge cuts
1 tablespoon balsamic vinegar

1 can diced tomatoes
4 cups water
1 tablespoon onion powder
1 tablespoon garlic powder
1 tablespoon paprika
1 teaspoon cayenne pepper
   (optional)

Directions

Add 4 cups of water and white beans to a saucepan.
Bring to a boil, reduce the heat, and let it simmer for 30 minutes.
Add all remaining ingredients.
Adjust the water if necessary.
Cook at low heat for another 30 minutes.
Turn off the heat, and serve immediately.

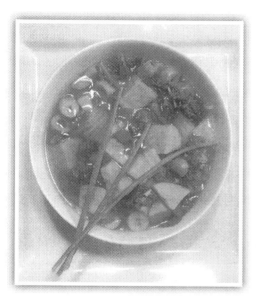

6. Broccoli Yammy Soup

Prep Time: 20 minutes
Yield: 3 servings

Ingredients
1 onion, diced
1 garlic clove, minced
2 yams, diced
1 cup broccoli florets
1 bunch bok choy, coarsely sliced
4 cups water
1 tablespoon onion powder
1 tablespoon garlic powder
1 tablespoon paprika
1 teaspoon cayenne pepper (optional)
1/4 cup green olives, sliced
1/4 cup dried tomatoes

Directions
Water-sauté onions and garlic in a pan until softened.
Add yams, broccoli florets, and bok choy.
Add 2 cups of hot water; bring to a boil.
Cook at low heat for 10 minutes.
Add all other ingredients plus the remaining 2 cups of water.
Simmer at low heat for another 10 minutes.
Turn off the heat, and serve immediately.

7. Black Forest Cream of Mushroom Soup (Dr. Fuhrman n.d.)

Prep Time: 40 minutes   Yield: 5 servings

Ingredients

2 tablespoons water
2 pounds mixed fresh
    mushrooms, sliced 1/4-inch
    thick
2 cloves garlic, minced or pressed
2 teaspoon herbs de Provence
5 cups carrot juice
3 cups unsweetened hemp, soy,
    or almond milk, divided
2 carrots, coarsely chopped
2 medium onions, chopped
3/4 cup fresh or frozen corn
    kernels
1 cup chopped celery

3 leeks, cut in 1/2-inch-thick
    rounds
1/4 cup no-salt seasoning blend,
    adjusted to taste
1/4 cup raw cashews
1 tablespoon fresh lemon juice
1 tablespoon chopped fresh
    thyme
2 teaspoons chopped fresh
    rosemary
3 cups cooked white beans, no
    salt added
5 ounces baby spinach
1/4 cup chopped fresh parsley, for
    garnish

Directions

Water-sauté mushrooms, garlic, and herbs de Provence for about 5 minutes, or until tender, adding more water if necessary to prevent from sticking. Set aside.

In a large soup pot, bring to a boil carrot juice, 2 1/2 cups of the nondairy milk, carrots, onions, corn, celery, leeks, and seasonings. Bring to a boil. Reduce heat and simmer until vegetables are tender.

In a blender, puree cashews and remaining 1/2 cup milk.

Add half of the soup liquid and vegetables, lemon juice, thyme, and rosemary. Blend until smooth and creamy.

Return pureed soup mixture to the pot.

Add beans, spinach, and sauté mushrooms.

Heat until spinach is wilted.

Garnish with parsley.

8. Kale and White Bean Soup (Sellani 2015)

Prep Time: 40 minutes   Yield: 6 servings

This hearty soup is packed with veggies and beans. A perfect meal for a cold winter evening.

Ingredients

2 carrots, diced

1 stalk celery, sliced in 1/8-inch-thick pieces

1 garlic clove, minced

1 large shallot, minced

4 tablespoons vegetable broth

1 can crushed tomatoes

2 cans water (use the empty tomato can)

3 cups kale, stems removed, cut into bite-size pieces

1 yam, peeled and cut into 1/4-inch-thick cubes

1 bay leaf

1/2 cup elbow macaroni (made from corn, gluten-free)

1 can navy beans, rinsed and drained thoroughly

1 teaspoon salt

1/2 teaspoon pumpkin pie spice

3–5 grinds of fresh black peppercorns

6 tablespoon pumpkin seeds

lemon for garnish (optional)

Directions

Heat vegetable broth in large soup pot on low temperature.

Sauté carrots, celery, garlic, and shallot in broth until soft.

Add canned tomatoes, water, and bay leaf. Bring to a boil.

Add kale and yam. Reduce heat to medium, keeping a slow boil.

Cook for an additional 10 minutes, until yam is just soft.

Add pasta and cook until tender.

Add beans, salt, pepper, and pumpkin pie spice.

Cook for another 2 minutes.

Discard bay leaf, and serve.

Top each bowl with 1 tablespoon pumpkin seeds and 1/2 slice of lemon.

9. New England Clamless Chowder (Rohrbacher 2015)

Prep Time: 70 minutes   Yield: 8 servings

Ingredients

1 pound firm tofu, finely diced, resembling clams format

1 large sweet onion, diced

2 celery stalks, diced

2 carrots, diced

1/2 cup garlic, chopped

1/2 pound cremini mushrooms, roughly chopped

1/4 cup white wine

1 tablespoon fresh thyme, chopped

2 teaspoon fresh or dried marjoram, chopped

6 cups no-salt-added or low-sodium vegetable broth

1 1/2 pounds fresh or frozen kale, chopped

2 roasted red peppers, diced

1 sweet potato, diced

1 red potato, diced

2 cups fresh or frozen corn kernels

1/4 cup chopped fresh parsley

1/2 cup nutritional yeast

1/2 teaspoon freshly ground black pepper

lemon wedges (optional)

For the Chowder Stock

2 cups steamed cauliflower florets

2 cups unsweetened soy, hemp, or almond milk (plus additional to achieve desired consistency)

2 tablespoonss whole wheat flour

2 tablespoon sesame seeds

1/2 cup nutritional yeast

1/4 cup lemon juice

2 teaspoons onion powder

4 cloves garlic

1/2 teaspoon dry mustard powder

2 tablespoons kelp powder

1 tablespoon no-salt seasoning blend

Directions

Spread tofu pieces on a baking sheet.

Bake at 350ºF for 45 minutes, stirring every 15 minutes, until lightly browned and slightly crispy.

Set aside.

In a large covered soup pot, sauté onions, celery, carrots, garlic, and mushrooms in white wine until onions are translucent and lightly golden.

Add herbs and sauté for another minute.

Add vegetable broth, kale, red peppers, and potatoes.

Simmer, covered, until vegetables are tender.

Puree all of chowder stock ingredients in a blender until smooth.

Add chowder to the pot with the vegetables and simmer for 10 minutes, adding the corn about halfway through.

Adjust consistency by adding additional nondairy milk.

Stir in parsley, nutritional yeast, tofu, and black pepper.

Serve with lemon wedges.

10. Thai Veggie Chickenot-Coconut Soup

Prep Time: 40 minutes   Yield: 4 servings

Ingredients
4 ounces cellophane rice noodles
6 cups low-sodium veggie broth
1–2 red thai peppers, seeded and finely chopped (plus slices for garnish)
3 cloves garlic, chopped
1 tablespoon grated ginger
2 tablespoons grated lemon zest
1 teaspoon grated lime zest
1/4 cup fresh lemon (or lime) juice
1/2 pound shiitake mushrooms, sliced
2 cups So Soy protein slices, soaked in water for about 15 minutes
1 cup light coconut milk
2 cups baby spinach
2 tablespoons chopped parsley (plus sprigs for garnish)

Directions
Place noodles in a bowl. Add enough warm water to cover, and let sit until soft. Drain.
Combine broth, pepper, garlic, ginger, lemon zest, lime zest, and lemon juice in a medium saucepan. Bring to a simmer.
Add noodles, and cook for 3 minutes.
Using tongs, transfer noodles to a bowl, and cover with foil to keep warm.
Add mushrooms to broth; simmer for another 3 minutes.
Add soy protein and coconut milk.
Simmer, stirring until soy protein is cooked.
Stir in spinach until it begins to wilt.
Add chopped parsley.
Using tongs, divide noodles among 4 bowls.
Ladle soup into bowls, and garnish with sprigs of parsley and slices of pepper.

11. Vegan Consommé

Prep Time: 90 minutes   Yield: 4 servings

Ingredients
1 cup soy protein, soaked in warm water for 15 minutes
1/4 can crushed tomatoes
10 cups strong vegetable stock
6 teaspoons agar-agar powder

Mirepoix
4 onions, finely diced
2 carrots, finely diced
1 celery stalk, finely diced
1 sachet containing parsley stems, 1 crushed bay leaf, 1 clove, and 1 teaspoon peppercorns

Directions
Strain soy protein to stockpot.
Add mirepoix and tomatoes.
Add about 2 cups of cold stock.
Let it simmer until it reaches boiling point.
Gradually stir in the remaining vegetable stock, mixing well.
Add sachet.
Set the pot on moderately low heat, and let it simmer slowly for about 45 minutes, stirring occasionally.
Bring mixture to a boil. Remove from heat.
Dissolve the 6 teaspoons agar-agar powder in 1/2 cup of cold water.
Add it to the stockpot.
Move the pot back to lower heat, and continue to simmer slowly for about 5 minutes. Do not stir or disturb the raft that forms on top.
Let it set while agar-agar forms a thick gelatin raft.
Using a ladle, carefully strain the consommé through a china cup lined with several layers of cheesecloth.
Season to taste with salt.
Garnish as desired.

12. "Caldo Verde" Portuguese Kale Soup

Prep Time: 45 minutes   Yield: 6–8 servings

Ingredients
1 large onion, diced
2 garlic cloves, sliced
1 pound cremini mushroom, sliced in coin shape
6 medium potatoes, diced
8 cups cold water
1 pound kale or collard greens, stem removed, cut into fine slices
freshly ground black pepper, to taste, although the Portuguese are fond
of white pepper

Directions
Water-sauté half the onions and mushrooms until lightly browned. Remove
from heat, and reserve.
Water-sauté the remaining onions.
Add garlic, and cook for 2 minutes.
Add potatoes and water.
Bring soup to a boil.
Lower the heat, and let it simmer.
Cook until potatoes are soft.
When caldo verde is cool enough to handle, puree it using a wand blender.
Add greens and mushrooms.
Bring everything back to boil, reduce the heat, and simmer for 2 minutes.
Season with salt and pepper, if desired.
Ladle caldo verde into bowls, and garnish with the remaining slices of
mushrooms and kale slices.

13. Fun Last-Minute Soup

Prep Time: 20 minutes   Yield: 3 servings

Ingredients
1 onion, cubed
1/2 garlic head, each clove cut in half
1 sweet potato, skin on, diced
1 russet potato, skin on, diced
4 cremini mushrooms, cut in fours
1 bunch of kale, finely sliced, stems on
1 bunch of swiss chard, finely sliced, stems on
2 celery stalks, sliced
2 tablespoons sliced green olives
1 can artichoke hearts, each cut in half
4 cups of water
1 tablespoon curry powder
1 tablespoon paprika
1 teaspoon black pepper (optional)

Directions
Water-sauté onions and garlic until softened.
Add potatoes, mushrooms, and 1 cup of hot water. Simmer for 2 minutes.
Add remaining ingredients and 3 cups of water.
Cook at medium heat for 15 minutes.
Serve in a soup bowl. Enjoy!

Vegetable Dishes

The vegetable dishes described here are meant to represent the entrees we normally eat in our standard diet. I wish to stress that, ideally, salads should be the main dish and these vegetarian dishes should compliment the meal.

1. Banzo Kale

Prep Time: 15 minutes   Yield: 2 servings

Ingredients

1 onion, diced

1 pound of cremini mushrooms, sliced

1 can of unsalted garbanzo beans

1 bunch of kale, roughly sliced

Directions

Sauté onions in a nonstick pan until soft.

Add mushrooms, and cook for about 2 minutes.

Add garbanzo beans, and cook for another 5 minutes.

Add kale, and cook until it changes color.

2. Raw Zucchini Pasta with Meatless Tomato Sauce

Prep Time: 30 minutes   Yield: 2 servings

Ingredients

2 raw zucchinis

1 cup soy protein

2 cups hot water

1 tablespoon low-sodium soy sauce

1 tablespoon balsamic vinegar

1 large onion, diced

1 can diced tomatoes, no salt added

1 tablespoon paprika

1 tablespoon onion powder

1 tablespoon garlic powder

1 teaspoon black pepper

Directions

Cut off the ends of zucchinis and make noodles using a vegetable spiralizer, or use a simple vegetable peeler to slice thin, fettuccini-style noodles. Set aside.

Soak soy protein in a mixture of hot water, soy sauce, and balsamic vinegar. Mix well, and let it soak for 15 minutes.

Sauté onions in a nonstick pan until soft.

Add tomatoes and seasonings to the onions, and cook for about 2 minutes.

Add soaked soy protein to the veggies. Cook another 15 minutes.

Divide zucchini noodles in two plates. Top with sauce.

Serve and enjoy!

3.   Brown Rice with Mushrooms and Peas

Prep Time: 30 minutes   Yield: 2 servings

Ingredients

1 cup brown rice uncooked

2 cups warm water

1 onion, diced

1 pound of cremini mushrooms, sliced

1 tablespoon onion powder

1 tablespoon garlic powder

Directions

Sauté onions in a nonstick pan until soft.

Add rice and mushrooms, and sauté for about 2 or 3 minutes.

Add onion and garlic powder.

Add hot water, and bring the mixture to a boil.

Add peas, and mix well.

Partially cover with a lid, reduce the heat to low, and simmer for 15 minutes or until all water is absorbed.

Serve with a side of lentils and a green salad.

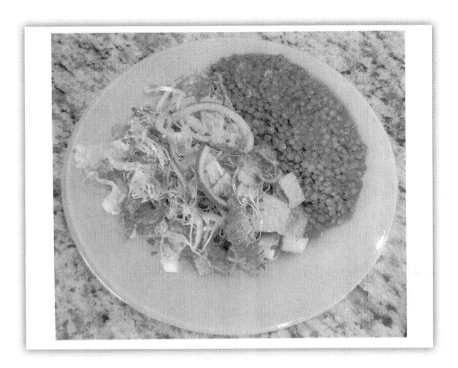

4. Simple Lentils

Prep Time: 15 minutes   Yield: 6 servings

Ingredients

1 cup brown lentils

3 cups water

1 tablespoon onion powder

1 tablespoon garlic powder

1 teaspoon white pepper

Directions

Combine lentils and water, and bring to a boil on high heat.

Add all seasonings. Reduce heat to low.

Partially cover pot with a lid, and simmer for 15 minutes.

Serve with brown rice and vegetables.

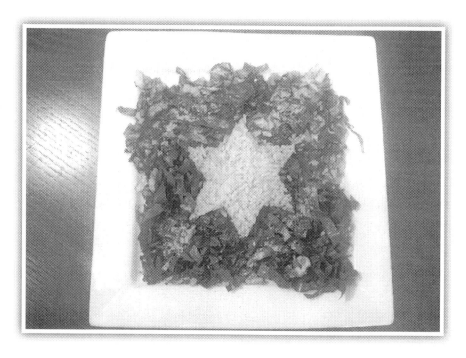

5. Collard Greens "a Mineira"

Prep Time: 15 minutes   Yield: 2 servings

Ingredients

4 bunches of collard greens
2 garlic cloves
1 tablespoon garlic powder

1 cup pecans
2 tablespoons nutritional yeast

Directions

Remove stems from collard greens.
Place them one on top of the other and then roll them up. Slice the roll as fine as you can. Reserve.
Sauté garlic in a nonstick pan.
Add collard greens and garlic powder.
Simmer for about 3–4 minutes.
Meanwhile, quickly heat the pecans until they release an aroma.
Add them to the collard greens, and mix well.
Top with nutritional yeast.
Serve it with rice or as a side dish.

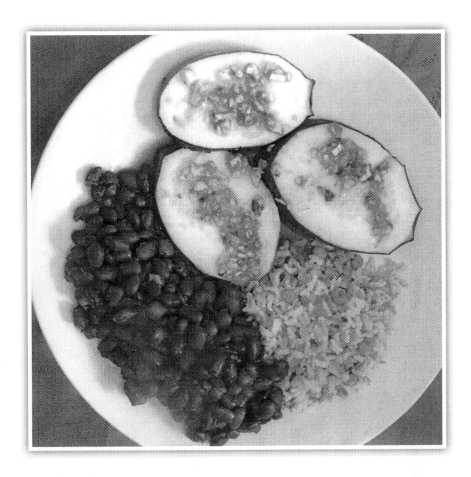

6. Grilled Zucchini

Prep Time: 15 minutes   Yield: 2 servings

Ingredients

2 large zucchinis
1 onion, finely diced
1 clove of garlic, finely diced
1 tablespoon low-sodium soy
   sauce

1 teaspoon liquid smoke
1 teaspoon chilli pepper
1 teaspoon of garlic powder
1 teaspoon of onion powder

Directions

Heat up the grill.

Mix all ingredients, except zucchini, to form a sauce.

Cut zucchinis into half-inch-thick slices.

Place zucchini slices on barbecue grill.

Top each slice with one spoon of the sauce mixture.

Grill for 5 minutes at medium heat.

Flip each slice.

Add sauce to the other side.

Grill for another 5 minutes.

Remove from the barbecue, being careful not to drop the sauce.

Serve with black beans and rice.

7.   Mushrooms with Daiya Cheese

Prep Time: 15 minutes   Yield: 2 servings

Ingredients

1 pound oyster mushrooms, roughly shredded

1 onion, diced

1/2 cup sliced green olives

1 teaspoon black pepper

1 teaspoon of garlic powder

1 teaspoon of onion powder

1/2 cup Daiya mozzarella cheese, shredded

Directions

Sauté onions in a nonstick pan until soft.

Add mushrooms, and cook for about 2 minutes.

Add green olives, garlic, and onion powder.

Add black pepper, and cook for another 5 minutes.

Add Daiya cheese, and cook until it melts.

Serve with rice and a salad.

8. Baked Cauliflower

Prep Time: 15 minutes   Yield: 2 servings

Ingredients
1 cauliflower head, separated in florets
1 onion, sliced
1 teaspoon of garlic powder
1 teaspoon of onion powder
1 cup toasted cassava flour
1/2 cup Daiya cheddar cheese, shredded

Directions
Preheat the oven to 375ºF.
Steam cauliflower florets with onion slices on top until soft.
Mix cassava flour with garlic and onion powder.
Sauté mixture of flour in a nonstick pan until golden.
Lightly oil a baking sheet.
Place florets in the baking sheet.
Top cauliflower florets with cassava flour mixture.
Add Daiya cheese.
Bake in the oven until cheese turns golden.
Serve with corn on the cob and a salad.

Note: Toasted cassava flour can be found in Brazilian or Portuguese grocery stores.

9. Eggplant Risotto

Prep Time: 40 minutes   Yield: 4 servings

Ingredients

1 eggplant, peeled and diced
3 garlic cloves, minced
4 cups water
1 small onion, minced
1 pound tomatoes, coarsely
    chopped
1 cup arborio rice

1/2 cup cold water
1 tablespoon tapioca starch
2 tablespoon nutritional yeast
1/2 cup julienned basil
salt, to taste (optional)
freshly ground pepper, to taste

Directions

Steam the eggplant and garlic until soft.

Remove from the heat.

In a large saucepan, sauté the onion and cook over moderate heat until softened.

Add all but 1/4 cup of the chopped tomatoes and cook, stirring, until softened.

Add rice. Cook, stirring until thoroughly coated.

Add 1 cup of the hot water. Keep stirring until water is nearly absorbed.

Continue adding hot water, 1 cup at a time, stirring until it is absorbed between additions.

The risotto is done when the rice is al dente and suspended in a creamy liquid.

Meanwhile, add the tapioca starch and nutritional yeast to one cup of cold water. Mix well to make a sauce.

Add tapioca sauce to the risotto. Mix well.

Cook for another 2 minutes.

Remove the risotto from the heat.

Add eggplant and basil to the risoto with the remaining 1/4 cup of tomatoes.

Season with pepper and transfer to bowls.

Serve immedietly.

10. Tofu Meatballs (Dr. Fuhrman n.d.)

Prep Time: 30 minutes   Yield: 4 servings

Ingredients
8 ounces firm tofu, drained
1/4 cup ground walnuts
1/4 cup rolled oats, blended to make coarse crumbs
2 tablespoons whole wheat flour
1 tablespoon dried parsley flakes
1/4 cup minced onion
1/2 teaspoon dried oregano
1/2 teaspoon dried basil
1 teaspoon low-sodium soy sauce

Directions
Mix all ingredients well, using hands if necessary.
Form into 2-inch balls.
Place on a baking pan that has been lightly oiled or lined with parchment paper.
Bake at 350ºF for 30–35 minutes or until golden.
Serve them topped with tomato sauce over zucchini pasta.

11. **Brazilian Black Beans** (Esselstyn plant-based diet recipes 2011)

Prep Time: 15 minutes   Yield: 6 servings

Ingredients
1 large onion, chopped
vegetable broth or water
2–4 garlic cloves, minced
1 tablespoon ginger peeled, grated, or minced
2 cans black beans, drained and rinsed
1 can diced tomatoes
1/4 teaspoon crushed red pepper flakes
cilantro or parsley, to taste

Directions
Water-sauté onion in a small amount of vegetable broth or water.
Add garlic and ginger, and stir-fry a few additional minutes.
Add beans, tomatoes, and pepper.
Simmer, stirring, 5–10 minutes, until heated through.

Chef's tip: For a quick and colorful meal, serve over brown rice surrounded by frozen peas rinsed in hot water. Or add corn, chopped bok choy, or other vegetables of your choice.

12. Farro Risotto with Spinach-Walnut Pesto and Roasted Tomatoes (Dr. Fuhrman n.d.)

Prep Time: 80 minutes   Yield: 5 servings

Ingredients

For the risotto
6 cups low-sodium or no-salt-added vegetable broth
1 1/2 cups farro
3 cloves garlic, chopped
1 shallot, chopped
1/2 cup dry white wine
10 plum tomatoes
1/2 teaspoon black pepper

For the Pesto
2 cloves garlic
1/2 cup walnuts
1/4 cup balsamic vinegar
1/2 cup water
1/2 tablespoon no-salt seasoning blend
1/2 tablespoon nutritional yeast
1 cup fresh basil leaves
4 cups fresh spinach

Directions
Heat broth to a simmer over medium heat.

Reduce heat to low, and keep warm.

Heat 2–3 tablespoons water in a large skillet, and sauté garlic and shallots until softened.

Add farro, and cook for one minute, stirring constantly.

Add wine; cook until all the wine is absorbed.

Add 1/2 cup hot broth, and cook until almost absorbed, stirring occasionally.

Continue adding broth in 1/2-cup increments, stirring occasionally for about 45 minutes or until farro is tender.

While farro is cooking, prepare the roasted tomatoes and pesto.

Preheat oven to 350°F.

Cut tomatoes lengthwise, and remove stem portion.

Place tomatoes cut side up on a rimmed baking pan that has been lightly wiped with oil.

Sprinkle with black pepper and roast for about 25 minutes or until tomatoes are soft and beginning to collapse.

To Make the Pesto

Blend garlic, walnuts, vinegar, water, seasonings, and nutritional yeast in a food processor.

Turn to low speed, and add basil and spinach, and pulse to a chunky consistency. Set aside.

Once farro is cooked, mix with desired amount of pesto, and serve with roasted tomatoes.

13. Raw Alkaline Alfredo (Tess 2015)

Prep Time: 10 minutes   Yield: 4 servings

Ingredients

For Raw Vegan Pasta Sauce
1 cup raw macadamias
1/2 cup raw pine nuts
3/4 cup filtered water
5 tablespoons freshly squeezed
    lemon juice
1 tablespoon finely chopped white
    onion
2 tablespoon cold-pressed, extra
    virgin olive oil
1 1/2 tablespoons finely chopped
    fresh garlic

1 teaspoon yellow mustard powder
1 teaspoon sea salt
1/2 teaspoon nutmeg

For Pasta Noodles and Assembly
8 zucchinis
2 cups cherry tomatoes sliced in half
2 cups broccoli, cut into tiny florets
1 cup finely chopped flat-leaf parsley
1/4 cup finely chopped spring onions
raw sesame seeds

Directions

To Make the Pasta Sauce
Place all sauce ingredients in a blender and puree on high until smooth and creamy.

To Make the Zucchini Noodles
Cut off the ends of the zucchinis and make noodles using a vegetable spiralizer or use a simple vegetable peeler to slice thin fettucine-style noodles.

To assemble
Add broccoli to pasta.
Toss sauce through the pasta with the broccoli.
Add most of the spring onions and parsley. Mix and season with salt to taste.
Swirl portions onto the middle of a plate.
Top with parsley and spring onions.
Surround with cherry tomatoes.

14. Wok-Seared Baby Bok Choy with Chili Oil and Garlic (Liano n.d.)

Prep Time: 20 minutes   Yield: 4 servings

Ingredients
1 tablespoon sesame seeds
4 heads baby bok choy
3 garlic cloves, thinly sliced
1/2 teaspoon red pepper flakes
1/4 cup low-sodium soy sauce
2 teaspoons Asian chili oil

Directions
In a small, dry frying pan over medium heat, toast the sesame seeds until golden brown and fragrant.
Transfer to a plate, and let cool.
Cut off the tough base from each head of bok choy.
Separate the heads into individual stalks by snapping the stalks away from their cores.
Heat a large fry pan over medium-high heat.
When the pan is hot and shimmering, add garlic and red pepper flakes.
Cook, tossing and stirring constantly, until fragrant but not browned, about 20–30 seconds.
Add bok choy and cook, tossing and stirring, until bok choy begins to wilt, about 1–2 minutes.
Add soy sauce and cook, stirring occasionally, until bok choy is tender and sauce evaporates, about 1–2 minutes.
Add chili oil, and stir well to coat bok choy. Remove from heat.
Add sesame seeds, and transfer bok choy to a warmed serving bowl. Serve immediately.

15. **Shiitake Broccoli Quiche** (Dr. Fuhrman n.d.)

Prep Time: 60 minutes   Yield: 8 servings

Ingredients

For the Piecrust
1 1/4 cups oat flour
3/4 cup raw cashew butter
5 tablespoons water

For the Filling
1/4 cup white wine
1 cup diced onion
2 cloves garlic, chopped
5 cups broccoli, cut into small florets
1 cup shiitake mushrooms, chopped
1 pound firm tofu, drained and squeezed
2 tablespoon raw cashew butter
3 tablespoon nutritional yeast
2 teaspoon dijon mustard
1 teaspoon mellow white miso
1 tablespoon shredded nondairy mozzarella
1 teaspoon dried basil
1/4 teaspoon nutmeg
1/8 teaspoon ground cayenne pepper, or to taste

Directions
Preheat oven to 350°F.

To Make the Crust
Place oat flour and nut butter in a bowl. Mash with a fork until crumbly.
Add the water one tablespoon at a time, and blend it with a fork.
Press dough evenly into a lightly oiled pie plate.
Bake for 10 minutes before adding filling.

To Make the Filling

Heat white wine in a medium saucepan over medium heat.

Add onions and garlic. Cook until softened, about 2 minutes.

Add broccoli. Cover and cook for 5 minutes, stirring occasionally and adding water as needed to prevent sticking.

Add mushrooms, and continue to cook until broccoli and mushrooms are tender.

In a food processor, blend the tofu and remaining ingredients until smooth.

Remove from blender, and combine with broccoli mixture.

Pour into the prebaked pie shell.

Bake for 30 minutes or until filling is thickened.

16. Southwestern Mac and "Cheese" (Sroufe 2013)

Prep Time: 50 minutes   Yield: 4 servings

Ingredients
1 medium yellow onion, peeled and diced
1 medium red bell pepper, seeded and diced
2 cups corn kernels (from about 3 ears)
1 jalapeño pepper, seeded and minced
2 teaspoons ground cumin
2 teaspoons ancho chili powder
salt, to taste
1 batch No-Cheese Sauce (see recipe 18)
1 can black beans, drained and rinsed
1/2 pound whole-grain elbow macaroni, cooked according to package directions, drained, and kept warm

Directions
Preheat oven to 350°F.
Saute onion and red pepper in a large saucepan, and sauté over medium heat. Add water 1–2 tablespoons at a time to keep the vegetables from sticking to the pan.
Add corn, jalapeño pepper, cumin, and chili powder, and cook for 30 seconds. Remove from heat, and season to taste.
Stir in the No-Cheese Sauce, beans, and cooked macaroni.
Spoon the mixture into a baking dish. Bake for 30 minutes or until bubbly.

Note: Macaroni and "cheese" gets a kick with corn, peppers, black beans, and spices.

17. No-Cheese Sauce (Sroufe 2013)

Prep Time: 5 minutes   Yield: 2 1/2 cups

Ingredients
1 large yellow onion, peeled and coarsely chopped
1 large red bell pepper, seeded and coarsely chopped
3 tablespoon cashews, toasted (optional)
1 tablespoon tahini (optional)
1 cup nutritional yeast
salt to taste

Directions
Combine all ingredients in a blender, in the order given, and puree until smooth and creamy.
Add up to 1/2 cup of water, if necessary, to achieve a smooth consistency.

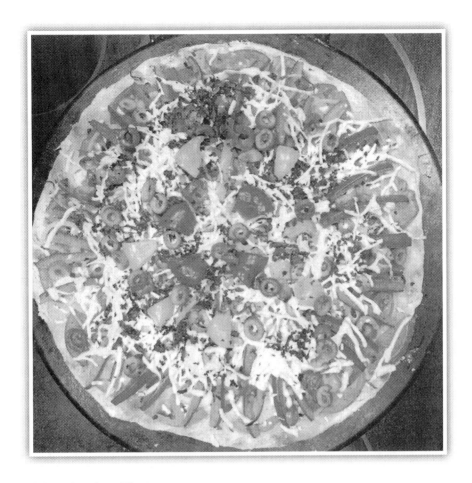

18. Garden Pizza

Prep Time: 45 minutes   Yield: 1 medium pizza

Ingredients

For the Dough

2 cups whole wheat flour
1 package rapid-dry yeast
1 cup warm water
2 tablespoons chia seeds

1/2 cup warm water
1 teaspoon salt
1 teaspoon sugar

For the Topping

2 red tomatoes, sliced
1 yellow tomato, sliced
1 green pepper, batonée

1/2 cup green olives
1 cup Daiya mozzarella cheese
1 cup spinach leaves

Directions

For the Dough

In a small bowl, dissolve yeast and sugar in warm water.
Let stand until creamy, about 10 minutes.
Blend chia seeds to make a meal, and let it soak in warm water for 15 minutes.
In a large bowl, combine 2 cups wheat flour, chia-seed mixture, salt, and the yeast mixture. Stir well to combine. Knead to form a dough.
Cover, and let it rise until doubled in volume.
Preheat oven to 350°F.
Lightly oil a pizza sheet.
Turn dough out onto a well-floured surface.
Form dough into a round, and roll out into a pizza-crust shape.
Bake for 20 minutes. Set it aside.

For the Topping

Spread slices of tomato over precooked dough.
Add a layer of spinach.
Add green pepper over the spinach.
Spread olives over the layer.
Sprinkle with Daiya cheese.
Decorate with yellow tomatoes.
Bake in preheated oven until golden brown.

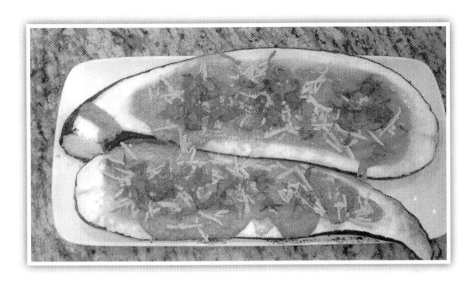

19. Baked Zucchini with Mushrooms and Green Olives

Prep Time: 45 minutes   Yield: 2 servings

Ingredients

2 large zucchinis, sliced
   lengthwise
1 onion, sliced
1 pound white mushrooms,
   sliced
1 cup green olives, sliced

1 cup low-sodium soy sauce
1 tablespoon onion powder
1 tablespoon garlic powder
1 teaspoon black pepper
1 tablespoon dry oregano flakes

Directions

Preheat oven to 375ºF.
Lightly oil a baking pan.
Spread zucchini slices to cover the bottom of pan.
Add a layer of onion slices.
Add mushrooms and olives
Make a sauce combining soy sauce and spices. Spread it over the layers.
Place remaining slices of zucchini on top.
Bake until golden.

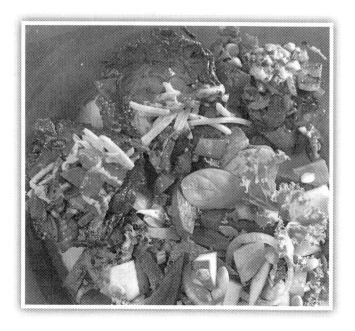

20.   Portobello Medallions with Daiya Cheese

Prep Time: 25 minutes   Yield: 4 servings

Ingredients
4 large portobello mushrooms, stems removed
4 tablespoons low-sodium soy sauce
1 teaspoon liquid smoke
1 tablespoon garlic powder
1 tablespoon onion powder
1 teaspoon cayenne pepper

Directions
Preheat oven to 375ºF.
Lightly oil a baking sheet.
Mix soy sauce and seasonings in a bowl.
Brush sauce over each mushroom cap, on both sides.
Place mushrooms upside down on baking sheet.
Bake for 15 minutes. Remove from oven.
Sprinle with Daiya cheese. Broil in oven for another 2 minutes.
Serve with a side of steamed vegetables.

Burgers and Sandwiches

I normally use leftover beans or lentils to make my burgers. When I season the beans ahead of time, I leave off part of the ingredients so they are not too spicy. You can always use canned beans instead; they work well and are very handy when there is no time to cook beans. I usually make sandwiches and wraps with any leftovers. They are very simple and easy to make.

1. Carrot Zucchini Burger

Prep Time: 15 minutes   Yield: 3 servings

Ingredientes
1 cooked potato, mashed
1 carrot, shredded
1 zucchini, shredded
1 cup green olives, finely
    chopped
1 cup cassava flour
1 cup oat flour
1 cup oatbran or bread crumbs
salt, to taste
1 cup finely chopped parsley
1 tablespoon onion powder
1 tablespoon garlic powder
1 teaspoon oregano
1 teaspoon curcuma

Directions
Combine vegetables in a bowl.
Add seasonings and olives.
Add cassava flour, and mix again.
If vegetables are too soft, add oatbran to adjust the consistency.
Make little balls, and mold each into a hamburger shape.
Dust with oatbran or cassava flour.
Grill or roast.

2. Black Bean Rice Burgers

Prep Time: 30 minutes   Yield: 2 servings

Ingredients

2 cups cooked black beans, drained

1 cup oats

2 cups cooked brown rice

2 tablespoons chia seeds

3 tablespoons warm water

2 onions, finely chopped

3 cloves garlic, minced

1 tablespoon low-sodium soy sauce

2 tablespoon tomato paste

1/2 teaspoon cumin

1/2 teaspoon liquid smoke

1/2 teaspoon smoked paprika

generous grating black pepper

Directions

Mix chia seeds and warm water in a small bowl. Set aside for 15 minutes.

Place beans and oats in a food processor, and pulse until they are finely minced.

Add chia seeds to the mixture, and pulse to combine well.

Add all remaining ingredients, and mix by hand.

Check consistency; if too soft, add oats to adjust.

Transfer mixture into a bowl. Set aside for about 15 minutes.

Preheat oven to 375ºF.

Line a baking sheet with parchment paper.

Shape burger mixture into 6 patties.

Place them on the prepared pan, and bake for about 30 minutes.

Remove patties from the baking sheet.

Serve at once or refrigerate for later use.

3. Savory Lentil-Mushroom Burgers (Voisin, *FatFree Vegan Kitchen* 2012)

Prep Time: 60 minutes   Yield: 6 servings

Ingredients

2 cups cooked lentils (green or brown), well drained
2 tablespoons chia seeds
3 tablespoons warm water
1 medium onion, finely chopped
6 ounces mushrooms, washed
3 cloves garlic, minced
1/3 cup old-fashioned oats
2 tablespoons potato starch or cornstarch
1 tablespoon low-sodium soy sauce
1 tablespoon tomato paste
1/2 teaspoon dried oregano
1/2 teaspoon dried basil
1/2 teaspoon smoked paprika
1/4 teaspoon dried thyme
generous grating black pepper

Directions

Cook 1 1/2 cups of lentils with dried thyme and black pepper in 3 cups of water for about 30 minutes.

Mix chia seeds and warm water in a small bowl. Set aside.

Place mushrooms into the food processor, and pulse until they are finely minced.

Heat a nonstick skillet over medium-high heat.

Add onions and cook until they begin to brown, adding a splash of water if they start to stick.

Stir in mushrooms and garlic; add another splash of water.

Cover, and cook until mushrooms soften (2–3 minutes), stirring often.

When mushrooms have softened, transfer them to the food processor, and add the lentils.

Pulse until lentils are combined with mushrooms.

Add chia-seed mixture and all remaining ingredients. Pulse to combine well.

Check consistency; if too soft, add oats to adjust.

Transfer mixture to a bowl. Set aside for about 15 minutes.

Preheat the oven to 375ºF.

Line a baking sheet with parchment paper.

Shape burger mixture into 6 patties.

Place them on the prepared pan, and bake for about 30 minutes.

Remove patties from the baking sheet.

Serve at once or refrigerate for later use.

4. BOMS Burgers (Dr. Fuhrman n.d.)

Prep Time: 15 minutes   Yield: 6 servings

Ingredients

1/4 cup sunflower seeds, chopped

2 medium portobello
   mushrooms, minced

3 cups cooked kidney beans

1/2 cup minced onion or shallots

2 tablespoons tomato paste

2 tablespoons ground flaxseeds

1–2 tablespoons rolled oats, as
   needed to adjust consistency

1/2 teaspoon chili powder or to
   taste

1 teaspoon low-sodium soy sauce

3 tablespoons dried mushroom

3 cloves roasted garlic (optional)

Directions

Preheat oven to 350ºF.

Lightly oil a baking sheet, or use parchment paper.

Chop sunflower seeds in a food processor to a coarse meal. Transfer to a large mixing bowl.

Roughly chop portobello mushrooms, and then pulse them in the food processor to mince.

Add to mixing bowl along with the remaining ingredients.

Use a potato masher to combine everything, adding enough rolled oats to get a patty that sticks together without being too dry.

Using a large ice cream scoop, portion the burgers; then flatten them out with wet fingers to avoid sticking.

Place patties on baking sheet, and bake for 25 minutes.

Remove from oven. Let cool slightly until you can pick up each patty and compress it firmly in your hands to reform the burger.

Return patties to baking sheet, bottom side up, and bake for another 10 minutes.

5. **Vegan Big Mac Recipe** (Veggiefull.com 2012)

Prep Time: 40 minutes   Yield: 2 servings

Ingredients

Vegan Big Mac Sauce (1/2 cup)
1 small avocado
1/4 tablespoon water
1/4 teaspoon salt
1/4 tablespoon lemon juice
1 3/4 teaspoons brown sugar
2 teaspoons dijon mustard
1/4 tablespoon olive oil
1 1/4 teaspoons white vinegar
1 1/2 tablespoons french dressing
3 teaspoons pickle/gherkin relish
1/2 tablespoon finely minced white onion

Other
4 soft bread rolls (2 used for the whole roll and 2 used only for the bottom half)
8 slices gherkin, thinly cut
2 tablespoons minced white onion
1 cup thinly sliced iceberg lettuce
2 vegan cheese slices

Veggie Burger (4 patties)
1 yellow onion
2 cloves garlic
1 can chickpeas, drained
2 tablespoons tomato paste
1 tablespoon fresh lemon juice
2 1/2 cups tightly packed bread crumbs
2 tablespoons barbeque sauce
1 teaspoon salt
3/4 teaspoon freshly cracked black pepper

Directions

Big Mac Sauce

Add all the sauce ingredients, except for the minced onion and pickle relish, to a blender. Blend until combined.

Add minced onion and pickled relish. Set aside.

Veggie Patties

In a food processor, add all veggie burger patty ingredients, and process until roughly combined.

Divide mixture into four parts and roll each into a well-combined ball.

Flatten the balls with your hands as flat as you can make them.

Lightly brush your grill with oil.

Grill each patty until browned and crispy on the outside.

Flip and grill the other side. Set them aside.

Cut 2 bread rolls in half. Set aside.

With the two remaining bread rolls, cut them in half and discard the top layer. Keep the two bottom layers for the middle layer of your final burgers. You will have two top layers and four bottom layers to use.

Assemble the Burger

Add one bread roll base layer to a plate.

Top bread with big mac sauce, lettuce, one slice of cheese, one veggie patty, minced onion, and two pickle slices.

Add another bread bottom layer.

Top with big mac sauce, lettuce, one veggie patty, minced onion, and two pickle slices.

Add the top of the bun.

6. Eggless Salad Sandwich

Prep Time: 10 minutes　　Yield: 2 servings

Ingredients
1 pack extra-firm organic tofu
1 tomato, sliced
1 lime, juiced
3 scallions, finely chopped
10–12 pitted olives
4 slices of whole grain bread
4–6 leaf lettuce
1 teaspoon garlic powder
1 teaspoon turmeric
4 teaspoons nutritional yeast
1 teaspoon mild yellow curry powder
sea salt and pepper, to taste

Directions
Drain and completely dry tofu.
Combine tofu with turmeric, garlic powder, nutritional yeast, and curry.
Mix well.
Add scallions, olives, and lime juice.
Lightly toast bread slices.
Place a lettuce leaf on a bread slice.
Place tofu mixture on top of lettuce.
Add a tomato slice.
Top with another bread slice.
Serve with olives on the side.

7. **Barbecue Pulled Jackfruit Sandwich** (Chow 2008)

Prep Time: 60 minutes to a day   Yield: 2 servings

Ingredients

1 can young green jackfruit in brine
2 cloves garlic, smashed
1 tablespoon olive oil
1/2 cup barbecue sauce, bottled or homemade
2 hamburger buns

Directions

Drain and wash the jackfruit in several changes of water.
After washing, squeeze out as much water as you can.
In a pan, heat oil and sauté garlic.
Add jackfruit; salt to taste. Cook for a 3–4 minutes over medium heat.
Transfer jackfruit to a slow cooker.
Add barbecue sauce, and mix well.
Set cooker for one hour, occasionally stirring and adding more sauce or water as needed.
Jackfruit should be fork-tender and come apart easily. Take jackfruit out of the cooker, and shred with a fork.
Let jackfruit sit for several hours or overnight to further develop flavor.
Serve on toasted buns with your choice of sauce, mayo, coleslaw, or pickles.

Desserts, Breads, and Cakes

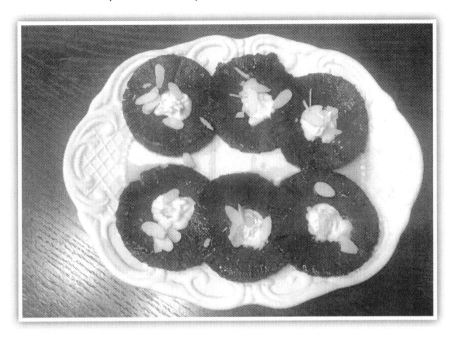

1. Red Wine Pineapple

Prep Time: 20 minutes   Yield: 15 slices

Ingredients

1 pineapple, peeled and cut in 15
   thin slices
1 cup sweet red wine

1 teaspoon cloves
2 cinnamon sticks

Directions

Heat a saucepan at high heat for about 30 seconds.
Add slices of pineapple to heated pan.
Add clove buds and cinnamon sticks.
Cook the pineapple in its juice, being careful not to let it overcook or burn.
Add wine once pineapple is cooked.
Cook the pineapple and wine for another 10 minutes over low heat.
Allow to cool and refrigerate. Serve cold.

2. The World's Healthiest Apple Pie (Voisin, *FatFree Vegan Kitchen* 2014)

Prep Time: 75 minutes   Yield: 4–6 servings

Ingredients

Crust
1 1/4 cups gluten-free oats
1/4 cup ground flaxseeds
1 teaspoon apple pie spice or cinnamon
4 ounces sulfite-free dried apples
8 ounces pitted dates
1 tablespoon alcohol-free vanilla extract

Filling
3 pounds apples
1 cup date paste
4 tablespoons lemon juice
4 tablespoons chia seeds
1 tablespoon alcohol-free vanilla
1 tablespoon apple pie spice or cinnamon
1/4 cup unsweetened coconut

Directions
Preheat oven to 350°F
Grind oats and seeds in a blender.
Transfer to a food processor fitted with an S blade.
Add spices and dried apples. Process until finely ground.
Add dates, a few at a time. Process until mixture starts to stick and you can clump it together easily into a ball.
Add vanilla, and briefly process again.
Evenly press mixture into a 9-inch springform pan.
In a small bowl, mix chia seeds and lemon juice. Set aside.
Peel apples and chop finely.
In a large bowl, add apples, date paste, spices, and vanilla.
Add chia seed / lemon juice mixture, and mix well.
Pour evenly over crust. Sprinkle with coconut.
Bake at 350°F until coconut starts to brown.

3. Pear Whipped Cream (AJ n.d.)

Prep Time: 20 minutes   Yield: 4 servings

Ingredients
1 can of pears in their own juice
1/3 cup raw cashews
1 tablespoon alcohol-free vanilla extract
1 teaspoon xanthan gum

Directions
Drain pears, and reserve juice for another use.
In a blender, blend pears until smooth.
Add remaining ingredients, and blend until incorporated.
Chill. Serve over fruit desserts.

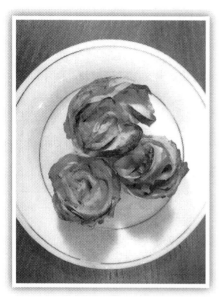

4. Apple Baked Roses
(Manuela 2015)

Prep Time: 90 minutes
Yield: 6 servings

Ingredients
4 apples, skin on, cored, and halved
2 cups water
1/2 lemon, juiced
3 pitted dates
2 tablespoon water
1 sheet of puff pastry
cinnamon powder, to taste

Directions
Preheat oven to 375ºF.
Add apples and two cups of water to a saucepan.
Cook apples until lightly softened. Set aside.
Add dates to a blender with 2 tablespoons of water. Blend to form a soft sauce. Set aside.
Flour your board, and roll out the puff pastry enough to make 6 strips, each 3 inches wide.
Score and cut dough with a pizza wheel or a knife.
Spoon out date sauce in the center of a strip of puff pastry.
Place apple slices in a row side by side overlaping each other on the strip of pastry, leaving the skin side of each apple along the edge of the dough.
Keep adding slices until you reach the end of the strip.
Fold the bottom part of puff pastry over the lower edge of apple slices.
Roll up puff pastry, making a shape like a rose.
Place roses in a greased baking sheet.
Bake for 35–45 minutes. Let it cool for 5 minutes.

5. Cocoa Truffles with Green Banana Biomass

Prep Time: 75 minutes   Yield: 10 truffles

Ingredients

1 cup green banana biomass (see Basic Recipes)
1 bar dark chocolate
1 teaspoon stevia sweetener
2 ounces dark chocolate, slivered

Directions

Melt chocolate bar in a double boiler.
Mix chocolate and stevia with banana biomass.
Form a smooth, homogeneous mixture. Use the mixer if necessary.
Refrigerate for 1 hour; then remove from fridge.
Use a spoon to scoop mixture, and roll into small balls.
Add slivered chocolate to a small bowl.
Roll each ball until fully coated by the chocolate.
Place each ball in a mini baking paper cup.

6. Orange Flan

Prep Time: 20 minutes   Yield: 2 servings

Ingredients

3 cups freshly squeezed orange juice
3 tablespoons stevia powder
3 tablespoons cornstartch
1/2 cup of cold water

Directions

Bring orange juice and stevia to a boil.
Dissolve cornstarch into cold water. Mix well.
Add cornstarch mixture to boiling orange juice, stirring constantly until thickened.
Simmer for 5 minutes.
Pour into a small serving bowl. Allow to cool, and place in the refrigerator for 3–4 hours.
Serve cold.

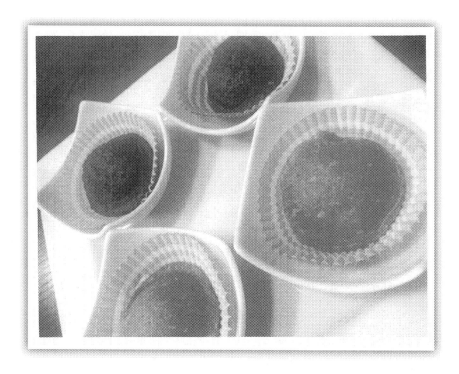

7. Vegan "Quindim"

Prep Time: 60 minutes   Yield: 24 quindims

Ingredients
1 cup coconut milk
1 1/2 cup agave syrup for yellow quindim or 1 1/2 cup black molasses for brown quindim
3 tablespoons soy milk powder (optional)
1/4 cup water
2 tablespoons coconut oil
3 tablespoons corn starch
3 cups raw cassava, grated
1/2 cup grated coconut
1 pinch saffron

Directions

Preheat oven to 350ºF

Add all ingredients, except grated coconut, to a blender.

Blend to a smooth consistency.

Transfer mixture to a bowl. Add grated coconut, and mix with a spoon.

Grease eight small ramekins. Pour an equal amount of the mixture into each one.

Bake in water bath for 40 minutes.

Let it sit until it cools. Remove from the ramekin, and enjoy.

8. Wine Sago Pudding

Prep Time: 2 hours 30 minutes   Yield: 10 servings

Ingredients
1 cup small tapioca pearls
6 cups water
2 cups red wine
1 cup stevia powder

Directions
Soak tapioca pearls in four cups of water for 2 hours.
Add tapioca pearls to water, wine, and stevia in a saucepan.
Cook over low heat, stirring constantly, until tapioca pearls become transparent.
Remove from heat. Allow to cool; then refrigerate.
Serve chilled.

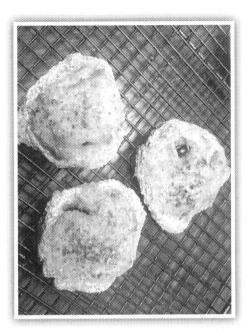

9. Cassava Rolls

Prep Time: 40 minutes
Yield: 15 rolls

Ingredients
2 cups cooked cassava root, mashed while still hot
8 tablespoons whole wheat flour
2 teaspoons chia seeds
2 tablespoons warm water
1 teaspoon cayenne pepper (optional)
1/2 cup nutritional yeast
15 black olives, sliced
dried oregano

Directions
Preheat the oven to 375ºF.
Using a food processor, grind chia seeds.
Mix the water and chia-seed meal in a bowl.
Allow to sit for 15 minutes.
Mix all ingredients together in a bowl to form a sticky dough.
Lightly oil a baking sheet.
Form small rolls, one at a time.
Add olive slices to the roll; top with dried oregano.
Place individual rolls unto the baking sheet, and flatten them a little.
Bake for 20 minutes or until golden.
Flip them, and bake for another 5 minutes.
Serve as snacks or a side dish.

10. Shirley's Bread

Prep Time: 2 hours 30 minutes   Yield: 1 loaf

Ingredients

2 tablespoons chia seeds

2 cups water

3 cups corn flour

1/2 cup amaranth flour

1 cup sour tapioca starch

5 capsules safflower oil

1 tablespoon agar-agar

1 tablespoon dry yeast

1 cup water

1 teaspoon salt

Directions

Soak chia in water until it forms a gel-like substance, about 15 minutes.

Add all dry ingredients to a large bowl, and mix.

Remove safflower oil from capsules. Add to the mix.

Add chia-seed gel.

Knead to form a dough. Add water if needed.

Continue to knead for about 10 minutes.

Place dough in a bread pan.

Let it rise for about 60 minutes.

Bake for 60 minutes.

11. White Corn Cake

Prep Time: 60 minutes   Yield: 8 servings

Ingredients

1/2 cup unsweetened applesauce

2 cups white corn flour

2 cups almond milk

3 tablespoons chia seeds

1 cup warm water

1 tablespoon baking powder

salt, to taste

Directions

Preheat oven to 375ºF.

Lightly oil a pudding baking pan.

Combine all ingredients in a bowl.

Mix well to incorporate all ingredients.

Place mixture in baking pan.

Bake for 35 minutes or until dry.

12. Gluten-Free Ciabatta (Estar 2014)

Prep Time: 50 minutes   Yield: 8 ciabattas

Ingredients

1 cup tapioca starch

1/2 cup of cassava root, cooked

2 tablespoons sour tapioca starch

1 tablespoon brown rice flour

1 teaspoon green banana biomass
    (see Basic Recipes)

2 tablespoons sunflower oil

1 tablespoon dry yeast

1/2 teaspoon sea salt

1/2 cup water

1 teaspoon coffee

2 tablespoons sunflower oil

Directions

Cook cassava root until soft, and mash it. Set aside.

Preheat oven to 375ºF.

Lightly oil a baking sheet.

Mix all dry ingredients.

Add liquid ingredients and mashed cassava.

Blend until the mixture is smooth and sticky.

Soak your hands in the water, and mold each ciabatta by placing it on the baking sheet.

Let ciabattas rise until doubled in volume.

Combine coffee and oil in a small bowl.

Brush each bread with the coffee-and-oil mixture.

Bake until the dough is golden.

13. Marble Cake

Prep Time: 45 minutes   Yield: 8 servings

Ingredients

White Dough
2 cups whole wheat flour
1 cup brown sugar or any
    sweetener of your choice
1/2 cup unsweetened applesauce
1 1/2 cups oat milk

1 teaspoon baking powder
1 teaspoon vanilla extract
1 tablespoon green banana
    biomass

Dark Dough
2 cups whole wheat flour
1 cup brown sugar or other
    sweetener of your choice
1/2 cup unsweetened green
    apples

1/4 cup cocoa powder
1 1/2 cups water
1 tablespoon baking powder
1 tablespoon green banana
    biomass

Filling
1 cup green banana biomass
5 dates
2 tablespoons cocoa powder
4 tablespoon hot water

Directions
Preheat oven to 375ºF.
Prepare white and dark dough in two separate bowls.
Add all ingredients for white dough. Mix well. Set aside.
Add all ingredients for dark dough. Mix well. Set aside.
Lightly oil a baking pan.
Add white dough to baking pan.
Place dark dough on top. Lightly swirl with a spatula.
Bake until dough is dry.

Festive Dishes for Special Occasions

1. Seitan Wellington

Preparation time: 1 hour 40 minutes   Yield: 6 servings

Ingredients

Stuffing

1/2 large onion, chopped
1 celery stalk, chopped
4 ounces mushrooms, sliced or
    chopped
1 teaspoon dried thyme

1/2 teaspoon rubbed sage
1/2 teaspoon black pepper
1 tablespoon soy sauce
1/2 cup water (more as needed)

Seitan

2 cups vital wheat gluten
1/4 cup nutritional yeast
1 teaspoon dried thyme
1 teaspoon rubbed sage
1 teaspoon marjoram
1 teaspoon cumin
1 teaspoon liquid smoke

1/3 can tomato sauce
1 tablespoon chia seeds or
    ground flaxseeds
1 1/2 cup vegetable broth
2 tablespoons soy sauce
1 clove garlic, peeled

Assembly

3 leafs vegan filo dough
3 tablespoon coconut oil
    (optional)

2 tablespoons almond milk
4 sprigs fresh rosemary

Directions

Stuffing

Water-sauté onion and celery.
Add mushrooms, thyme, sage, and black pepper. Cover with a lid.
Cook over medium heat until mushrooms exude their juices.
Add remaining ingredients.
Add enough water to moisten stuffing but not make it soaking wet.
Remove from heat. Keep covered.

Make Seitan

In a mixing bowl, combine all dry ingredients.

Blend 1 1/2 cups of broth, soy sauce, and garlic in blender until liquefied.

Make a hole in the center of the dry ingredients, add blended mixture, and stir until gluten is completely moistened.

Knead dough until it holds together in a ball.

Preheat oven to 400°F.

Lightly oil an oval or rectangular baking pan. (Do not to use a wide pan.)

Place the dough in the center of baking pan.

Cover it with aluminum wrap.

Roll out the seitan, making sure that it is the same thickness in all places.

Bake for 30 minutes. Remove from oven; let it cool.

Assemble

Line your work surface with the 3 sheets of filo dough, one on top of the other.

For a fluffier dough, lightly brush coconut oil between layers.

Once seitan is cool, cut it in 6 even slices, but do not completely separate them from the whole piece.

Spread half of the stuffing evenly between each slice.

Spread a thin layer of the stuffing in the center of the filo dough.

Put the seitan with the stuffing on top of the stuffing layer in the filo dough.

Spread the remaining stuffing on top of seitan.

Lift up one side of filo dough, and bring it up along the edge of seitan to cover it. Do the same with the other side.

Pinch ends of dough sealed.

Make sure that all edges are completely sealed without any gaps or stuffing showing.

Lift the seitan roll carefully, and place it seam side up in the prepared casserole dish.

Lightly brush dough with almond milk. Spread rosemary over dough.

Cover tightly with aluminum foil. Bake for 25 minutes.

Remove from oven. Remove aluminun foil.

Baste with almond milk.

Return to oven uncovered for about 30 minutes.

Remove from oven. Let it cool for 5–10 minutes.

Transfer carefully to a cutting board or serving platter.

Separate precut slices to serve.

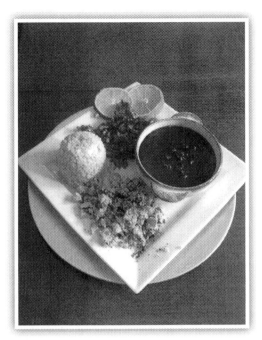

2. Brazilian "Feijoada" Quasi-Traditional

Preparation time: 1 hour 40 minutes
Yield: 6 servings

Ingredients
2 pounds black beans
4 pounds water
1 carrot, fine diagonal slices
1 beet, fine diagonal slices
1/2 pound smoked tofu, medium sliced
1 cup soy protein
1 soy sausage
1 garlic clove
1 onion, diced
2 bay leaves
1 cup parsley, finely chopped

Directions
Place beans in a large pot.
Add water, bay leaves, carrots, and beets.
Bring to boil over high heat.
Reduce the heat to low, and partially cover the pot.
Let it simmer for about one hour.
In a nonstick pan, sauté onions and garlic until soft.
Add tofu, soy protein, and sausage. Cook for about 5 minutes, mixing so it does not burn.
Add this mixture to the beans.
Simmer at low heat for about 1 hour, until beans are soft.
Add water if it is getting dry. It should be a coarse soup consistency.
Remove from heat. Add parsley.
Serve with brown rice, collard greens "à mineira," and orange slices.

Basic Recipes

The recipes below are a combination of plain ingredients that can be kept premade and available to use in some situations or recipes that call for them. Some may be stored in a freezer for up to three months; others are to be used within a couple of days. They are very handy and quite simple to make.

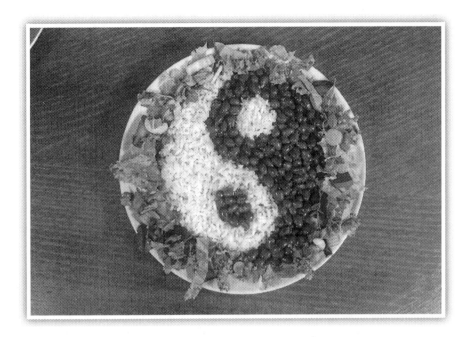

1. Dried Beans

Prep Time: 40 minutes   Yield: 2 portions

Ingredients

1 cup dried beans (any kind)   1 garlic, minced
2 liters water   1 teaspoon black pepper
1 onion, diced

Directions

Soak beans overnight. Strain and wash soaked beans.
Place beans and water in a large pot. Bring to a boil.
Reduce heat. Cook, partially covered, until soft.
Water-sauté onions and garlic.
Add a tablespoon of soft cooked beans to fry pan, and mash them to release starch.
Add black pepper.
Return mixture to bean pot.
Cook for a few minutes.
Serve over brown rice.

2. Brown Rice

Prep Time: 30 minutes   Yield: 3 portions

Ingredients
1 cup rice (or any other grain)
2 cups of hot water
1 onion, diced
1 clove garlic, minced
1 teaspoon onion powder
1 teaspoon garlic powder

Directions
Water-sauté onions and garlic.
Add rice and sauté for a few minutes.
Add hot water. Bring to a boil.
Reduce heat; cook, partially covered, until water is dry.
Serve with beans and vegetables.

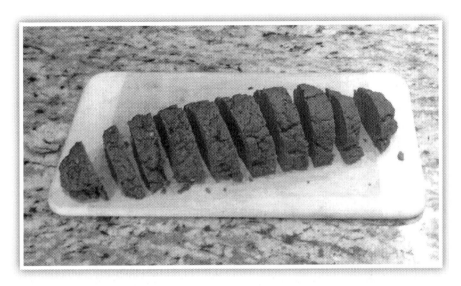

3. Seitan "Steak"

Prep Time: 45 minutes   Yield: 4–6 "steaks"

Ingredients

2 cups vital wheat gluten
1/4 cup nutritional yeast
1 teaspoon dried thyme
1 teaspoon rubbed sage
1 teaspoon marjoram
1 teaspoon cumin
1/3 can tomato sauce

1 tablespoon chia seeds or
    ground flaxseeds
1 1/2 cups vegetable broth
1 teaspoon liquid smoke
2 tablespoons soy sauce
1 clove garlic, peeled

Directions

In a mixing bowl, combine all dry ingredients.
Blend broth, soy sauce, and garlic in blender until liquefied.
Make a hole in the center of the dry ingredients, add blended mixture, and stir until gluten is completely moistened.
Knead dough until it holds together in a ball.
Cut dough in slices. Set aside.
Preheat oven to 400ºF.
Lightly oil a baking pan.
Place each steak in the baking pan.
Cover them with aluminum wrap.
Bake for 15 minutes.
Remove, and use as meat replacement.

4.   Oat Milk

Prep Time: 5 minutes   Yield: 1 liter

Ingredients
2 cups oat flour or flakes
4 cups water

Directions
Blend all ingredients. Strain.
Store in a glass bottle. Refrigerate. Use within 3 days.

5.   Green Banana Biomass

Prep Time: 40 minutes   Yield: 24 portions

Ingredients
6 green bananas (the greener the better)
2 liters water

Directions
Wash green bananas very well.
Place water in a pressure cooker, and let it boil.
When the water is boiling, add bananas to pressure cooker.
Place the lid on pressure cooker.
Cook for 8 minutes.
Turn off the heat.
Let pressure release naturally, about 15 minutes.
Remove bananas from water while hot.
Peel bananas, and place them in food processor.
Process to get a soft cream.
Place cream in an ice-cube tray.
Keep refrigerated for 3 days or in the freezer for up to 3 months.

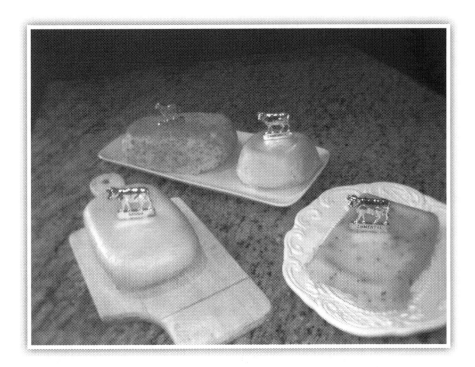

6.   Cassava Cheese

Prep Time: 40 minutes   Yield: 3 cheeses of 250 gr each

Ingredients
3 cups of cassava pureed as instructed below
1 cup sour tapioca starch (found in Portuguese supermarkets)
1 cup regular tapioca starch
2 cups of water
1/2 cup of sunflower oil
1/2 cup nutritional yeast
1 teaspoon salt or to taste
1/2 cup lemon juice

Directions

Cook cassava root in water for about one hour until soft but not falling apart remove the hard middle string from each piece and discard it.

Leave the cassava to cool in it's own water.

Separate cassava on from it's water and keep the water on the side.

Add 2 cups of cold cassava cooking water to a mixer.

Add 3 cups of cold cassava pieces to the mixer and puree it well.

Add all other ingredients in the mixer and mix it till achieving a smooth consistency.

Take this mixture to the stove in a large pan on low heat for about 5 to 8 minutes mixing it strongly until the dough becomes a firm ball. Do not allow it to boil.

Spread this mixture in a mold, weight each portion to 250 gr to form a "cheese".

Take cheeses to the fridge until they become hard, (about a day).

Use as a regular cheese up to two weeks in the fridge.

References

AJ, Chef. n.d. *UCD Integrative Medicine Program*. http://www.ucdintegrative medicine.com/recipes/the-worlds-healthiest-apple-pie/.

Anthony, Chef Mark. 2015. *Brand New Vegan*. 06 09. http://www. brandnewvegan.com/recipes/amazing-vegan-cheese-sauce/.

Campbell, T. Colin. 2004. *The China Study*. Dallas: BenBella Books, Inc.

—. 2013. *Whole: Rethinking the Science of Nutrition*. Dallas: BenBella Books, Inc.

2015. Center for Nutrition Studies. http://nutritionstudies.org/recipes/ salad/four-bean-salad/.

Cheeke, Robert. 2004. 10 11. http://www.veganbodybuilding. com/?page=article_proteincontent.

Chow. 2008. *Chow Vegan*. 05 28. http://chowvegan.com/2008/05/28/ bbq-pulled-jackfruit-sandwich/.

Colins, Sandy. 2015. *Nutritarian Recipe Page*. 10 26. https://www. drfuhrman.com/members/VwRecipe2.aspx?id=2191.

drfuhrman.com. n.d. *Dr. Fuhrman*. https://www.drfuhrman.com.

da Rosa, Marco Aurelio Camargo, Cristiano Mauro Assis Gomes, Neusa Sica da Rocha, Felix Henrique Paim Kessler, Sonia Maria Blauth de Slavutzky, Efigenia Ferreira e Ferreira, Flavio Pechansky. 2012. 02 14. http://www.scielo.br/scielo. php?script=sci_arttext&pid=S0102-79722013000100009.

Estar, Bem. 2014. *Cliquetando*. 05 15. http://cliquetando.xpg.uol.com. br/2014/05/ciabatta-sem-gluten-receita-bem-estar-15052014.html.

Fuhrman, Dr. 2005. "Cancer's stark realities." *Healthy Times*, 22 ed.

Fuhrman, Joel. 2011. "Eat to Live." In *Eat to Live: the amazing nutrient-rich program for fast and sustainable weight loss*, by Joel Fuhrman, 171. New York, NY: Brown and Little Company.

—. 2012. *Diabetes lifestyle intervention trial fails: Modest changes bring modest results.* 11 02. http://www.diseaseproof.com.

Iron rich foods for vegetarians and vegans. 2013. 02 01. http://bembu.com/iron-rich-foods-for-vegetarians-and-vegans.

Stanger, Janice, PhD. 2016. *The Perfect Formula Diet.* 03 16. http://perfectformuladiet.com/health/sugar-is-not-the-great-evil/.

Klaper, Michael. 2013. *Answers.* 08 18. www.docorklaper.com/answers/answers11/.

Krantz, Rachel. 2016. *Bustle.* 02 15. http://www.bustle.com/articles/137865-8-reasons-meat-is-bad-for-you-yes-even-chicken.

Leung, Andrew. 2016. *Science. Mic.* 03 17. http://mic.com/articles/138240/here-are-10-unexpected-high-protein-foods-that-aren-t-meat-or-tofu#.VVPfOX6OC.

Liano, Jodi. n.d. *Williams-Sonoma.* http://www.williams-sonoma.com/recipe/wok-seared-baby-bok-choy-with-chili-oil-and-garlic.html.

Manuela. 2015. *Quick and Easy Italian Recipes.* 03 26.

Montignac, Michel. n.d. *Montignac Methode.* http://www.montignac.com/en/the-history-of-man-s-eating-habits/.

Peto, Doll R. R. 1981. *Pub Med.* Accessed 12 10, 2015. www.ncbi.nlm.nih.gov/pubmed/7017215#.

Reuters. 2016. *Health Diet and Fitness.* 03 22. http://www.nbcnews.com/health/diet-fitness/vegan-eating-would-slash-cut-food-s-global-warming-emissions-n542886.

Ribeiro, Lair. 2013. *Dr Lair Ribeiro Agua com PH alto x refrigerante.* 06 23. www.youtube.com/watch?v=_NTU0tXcm8g.

Rohrbacher, James. 2015. *Dr Fuhrman's.* 02 11. https://www.drfuhrman.com/members/VwRecipe2.aspx?id=2377.

Sass, Cynthia. 2016. *Time.* 03 14. http://time.com/4257605/eat-more-vegetables/.

Sellani, Sandra. 2015. *Center for Nutrition Studies.* 08 12. http://nutritionstudies.org/recipes/soup/kale-white-bean-soup/.

Sofia Pineda Ochoa, MD. 2016. 03 19. http://www.forksoverknives.com/7-ways-milk-and-dairy-products-are-making-you-sick/.

Sroufe, Del. 2013. *Forks over Knifes.* Jan 28. http://www.forksoverknives. com/recipes/no-cheese-sauce/.

Success Stories. n.d. Accessed 06 21, 2011. https://www.drfuhrman.com/ success/success.aspx.

Sugar, Jenny. 2011. 08 11. http://www.popsugar.com/fitness/ Nutritional-Comparison-Tofu-Tempeh-Seitan-Recipes-18692390.

Tess. 2015. *The Blender Girl.* 07 17. http://healthyblenderrecipes.com/ recipes/raw_vegan_alfredo_pasta.

Vegetarian Times. 2011 11 13. http://www.vegetariantimes.com/recipe/ asparagus-with-vegan-hollandaise/.

2011. *Vegetarian Times.* 11 13. http://www.vegetariantimes.com/recipe/ asparagus-with-vegan-hollandaise/.

Veggiefull.com. 2012. 10 19. http://www.veggieful.com/2012/10/vegan- vegetarian-big-mac-recipe.html.

To Lower Cholesterol Naturally. 2011. *Natural Ways Of Lowering Cholesterol.* September 16. http://www.tolowercholesterolnaturally.com/ essylstyn-plant-based-diet-recipes-lower-cholesterol-with-diet/.

Vibrant Live Magazine. 2011. "Esselstyn plant based diet recipes." May/June.

Voisin, Susan. 2012. *FatFree Vegan Kitchen.* 09 12. http://blog.fatfreevegan. com/2012/09/savory-lentil-mushroom-burgers.html.

—. 2014. *FatFree Vegan Kitchen.* 09 14. http://blog.fatfreevegan. com/2014/09/miraclenaise-soy-free-mayo-plus-roasted-red- pepper-dressing.html.

W, Kaitlin. 2014. *Vegan Baking: Easily Replace Eggs in Your Favorite Recipes.* 06 05. http://www.swansonvitamins.com/blog/kaitlins-blog/ egg-substitutes.

Warinner, Christina. 2014. 06 19. http://www.singjupost.com/ debunking-paleo-diet-christina-warinner-transcript/.

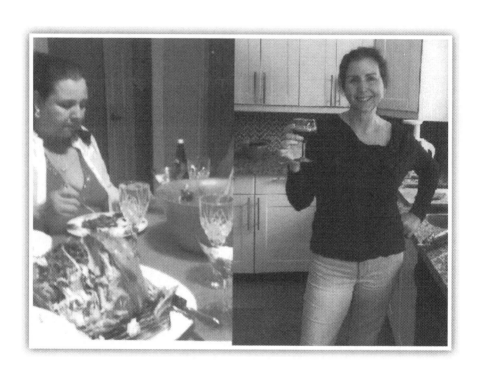

Index

W

Printed in the United States
By Bookmasters